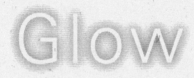

Glow

A Prescription for Radiant Health and Beauty

CHRISTINA PIRELLO

HPBooks

HP Books
Published by The Berkley Publishing Group
A division of Penguin Putnam Inc.
375 Hudson Street
New York, New York 10014

First edition: November 2001
Published simultaneously in Canada.

Visit our website at www.penguinputnam.com

Library of Congress Cataloging-in-Publication Data

Glow / Christina Pirello.
    p.   cm.
Includes index.
ISBN 1-55788-370-X
    1. Beauty, Personal. 2. Cookery (Natural foods) 3. Health—Nutritional aspects. I. Title.
RA784 .P56 2001
613.2—dc21   00-054131

PRINTED IN THE UNITED STATES OF AMERICA

20 19 18 17

To Olivia,
in whose eight-year-old face,
I see the hope and beauty of the world that is to come

Contents

Acknowledgments

No man (or woman) is an island and that is never more obvious to me than when I'm writing a book. There are so many people to thank for their help, wisdom, and support that it could be a book in itself. Don't panic; I'll be somewhat brief.

I'd like to thank Michael Potter, owner and president of Eden Foods, Inc. Michael, your fierce commitment to our shared vision and work toward improving and protecting the food we eat inspires me daily. Without your vision and generosity, much of what is known as "Christina Cooks" would be merely a dream.

I have the deepest gratitude to John Duff, my publisher and friend, for your confidence and support of my work. With your feet planted firmly in the real world, you keep me from "woo-woo land." And to Jeanette Egan, my editor, for all your hard work and commitment to keeping me real and accurate.

Thanks so much to Patrick Riley, my dear friend and shiatsu massage therapist, for your input into this book and for your magic touch. Your loving energy has brought me back into balance from the brink so many times that I have lost count.

I'd like to thank my many teachers, for sharing their wisdom with me and for the support and encouragement to find my own voice in my work. I'd especially like to thank Murray Snyder, for all that he taught me to see in the simple lines of the hand.

I could never express my gratitude to my students for continually allowing me access to their lives and for the honor of sharing with them what little I know. Through them, I am always drawn back to the beginner's mind. Thanks for keeping me humble and for teaching me so much.

I'd like to thank my family, but especially my big brother, Tom, the family genius, for the unconditional love and support that he gives me as I stumble through my life as a writer and performer, professions at which he is more adept.

To my precious girlfriends. Without you, I would have caved a long time ago. Thanks for your unwavering love, support, shoulders (for crying), ears (for listening to rants), eyes for proofreading, and tummies for experimental recipes. Your friendships are the greatest blessings in my life. You know who you are.

Finally, thanks to my hero . . . my partner, husband, and love of my life. Robert, your visions and dreams for us and for the world inspire me to be the best person I can be. Your integrity and strength of character are without compare and I know that I am safe with you. Thank you for your love and for being my soft place to fall.

Introduction

was born into a lusty Italian family, bursting with pas-
sionate emotion. To them—and therefore, to me, every man,
woman, and child was beautiful. Whether their cheeks were soft and
dewy or lined with the wisdom that comes with age, I was taught to
see not only their outer beauty, but also their inner radiance.

We live in a world obsessed with beauty, so much so, that we are
bereft at the lack of it. We drink it in, intoxicated by its power. We
crave it and bask in its light. However, somewhere along the way, we
lost the vision of true beauty, and instead worship in its place, artificial,
applied beauty.

My childhood vision of beauty, my eye trained by my grandfather,
has never changed. I marvel at all natural beauty, from a sweeping landscape to a simple pot of begonias blooming on a city stoop; from a
beautiful baby to a weathered, wise face. And while I am as enchanted
as anyone by perfect skin, lustrous hair, clear eyes, and chiseled features,
the beauty that inspires me is the beauty that is intangible—that glow
that comes from within—when a person is joyously happy, fulfilled in
their work, content with themselves, and vital with health.

When I was a child, I didn't know what created the glow that I so admired and continue to admire today. I never understood the concept of beauty from the inside. My own health crisis, which brought me to the study of whole foods cooking and traditional healing arts, provided me with the answers I craved. My study of the energy of food and natural harmony unlocked many of life's mysteries. I learned that gratitude and contentment with life create more beauty than any hair dryer.

Our current view of beauty often involves perfection of features and is unattainable by most of us. Beauty isn't the perfect shade of lipstick or the finest suit or the perfect size waist or length of leg. It's not about blue eyes or perfect teeth. Those things are just the icing on the cake. And while lovely to see, these features are not the heart of true beauty.

If we're truly honest with ourselves, we'll admit that when we aren't feeling well and vital, no amount of makeup or hair gel shores up our confidence. We skulk through the day, praying for the moment when we can crawl into bed and hopefully wake on a higher note. But on those mornings when we feel marvelous, a light swish of the mascara wand or fingers carelessly run through our hair and we bound out of the house, ready to face the day, feeling confident, graceful, beautiful, handsome, and glowing.

I've learned a lot in my studies and in my work about the effect of food on our bodies and its power over our health. My own experience with transformation has taken me from obesity, oily skin and hair, struggles with blemishes, freckles, and excessive body hair to a life virtually free of those challenges. Hindsight is indeed 20/20 and in my own view of my life, I see where I misstepped, over and over. I now know that it is truly our birthright to look beautiful and feel well and it is in our choices that we forfeit that right, creating the never-ending struggle to regain it, as only we can.

And so I have created this book, delving into the world of traditional healing practices and Chinese medicine. With it, I hope that you will come to understand your strengths and weaknesses and nourish them both to regain your balance, internally and externally. Understanding what we eat is a key factor in creating our health and our health is a key factor in our appearance. Once you've mastered that, the path to glowing, radiant beauty is straight and true. Season to season, age to age, the face and form you present to the world will be strong, vital, and stunningly beautiful.

I wish you health, beauty, and a long and happy life, filled with gratitude, joy, strength, and abundance.

Glow

Your Glowing Roots

Radiance, beauty, that "glow" are the elusive states of being that we all seek to achieve. I would venture to say that many would rather look good than feel good. Unfortunately, you can't have one without the other. Like love and marriage, looking great is usually the result of feeling great, and conversely, if you don't feel well, it's hard to put your best face forward.

Every year, *People* magazine issues its list of the fifty most beautiful people in the world, and while some of them are exquisite, some are hardly what we would call classically beautiful. There is one common denominator among all these faces, however, a factor that makes people attractive and beautiful, whether famous or not, classically or not. If you were to analyze what is truly attractive, I think you would surprise yourself when you discovered that it wasn't really his blue eyes or her long legs, but their "glow." People that we deem beautiful are brimming with vitality. And that vitality allows them to walk with a straight, confident stride, head held high. That vitality is what creates their perfect skin and lustrous hair and is what we find so attractive. We are attracted to health. We want to be near it and bask in its radiance.

Beauty isn't limited to surface appearance. It is the total sum of being. There are no absolute standards by which we judge beauty. It truly is in the eyes of the beholder, with each culture varying its concept of what is considered attractive. And while beauty changes from culture to culture and even season to season, with what's "in" and "out," what never changes is the fact that beauty is dynamic and whole, not the fragments of an image.

It is our birthright to be beautiful. By that, I mean that it is our nature to be healthy, to be our very best selves. That natural, radiant glow comes from within and is not the result of artificial application of cosmetics to mask the truth. Our beauty, or lack thereof, is a simple reflection of our day-to-day life. Elegance, grace, and beauty arise naturally from good health, with little need for enhancement or artifice. Our glow is from within, rather than purchased and applied.

The word *cosmetics* has its roots in the Greek word *cosmos*, a word used to describe the order of nature. By classic definition, to be beautiful was to be in harmony with nature. Beauty, therefore, is a reflection of natural harmony.

The approach to natural, radiant beauty and health that I take in this book is based on a holistic and comprehensive understanding of the order of nature and our place within our environment. It is only with understanding of life and its energy that we can achieve our dreams and goals.

There are many factors that influence our natural, radiant health. Remember that the body is an interconnected being, not simply a collection of parts. Problems with the skin, hair, nails, and overall appearance are clear reflections of internal conditions and no amount of lotions, potions, creams, oils, shampoos, rinses, or powders will solve the internal dilemmas causing the complaints. They will simply mask the symptoms; the disorder will continue and the symptoms will perpetuate. We will spend more money and grow more despondent over our deteriorating appearance.

To achieve our own natural radiant glow, we must begin to understand the relationship between our internal and external conditions. As we grow more aware of the connection between health and vital beauty, we can begin to realize that our appearance is a reflection of our daily life, from our food choices, to exercise and activity, to our environment, to our attitudes and emotions. As with health, our natural, radiant glow is something that we create daily, through the choices that we make.

Achieving naturally radiant beauty is actually quite simple, requiring only a balanced diet, proper activity and a positive self-image. It really doesn't require expensive spa treatments (although they are a lovely indulgence to be enjoyed on occasion) or the expenditure of large sums of money for products to simulate the look we so desperately seek. By simply making choices appropriate to us, as humans, we can achieve the radiant health and beauty that is ours by virtue of who we are.

The Source of Radiance

The approach to radiant health and beauty that I present in this book is based on a holistic and comprehensive view of the human body. In contrast to the modern approaches that deal with surface appearance, my approach considers underlying influences that result in the surface appearance. The body is an interconnected whole, not a collection of unrelated parts and so to affect external symptoms, we must consider the internal imbalances that may have contributed to our condition.

Each day, people grow more aware of the connection between health and diet. In the same manner, we must embrace the idea that, like health, natural radiance is something that we create in our day-to-day lives. Achieving natural beauty is quite simple. The only "tools" required are a balanced diet, exercise, daily grooming, natural body care, and a positive attitude. Understanding the power of our daily choices produces the results we crave. We must realize that when we balance our bodies with nature, a beautiful, radiant appearance is ours, the result of the foods we choose to eat, the activities we pursue, and the way we see the world around us.

Each of us exists in an environment and our interaction with that environment contributes to the creation of humanity. As we all are aware, clean, natural surroundings are essential to life. Clean air to breathe, clean water for drinking, bathing and cooking, sunlight, lush green vegetation, and a peaceful setting create an environment in which natural radiance is easier to achieve. We have a certain degree of control over these factors with our choices in living space, leisure activities, our jobs and our understanding of how humanity impacts nature. However, the environmental factor over which we have the most control is our daily choice of food.

Food is simply a condensed version of our larger environment and is the material that nature uses to construct our human bodies. Minute to minute, second to second, new cells, muscles, tissue, body fluids, and bone are being created or affected by what we choose to eat and drink. We are, in many ways, the creation of what we put in our mouths every day. Our health, radiance, and beauty (or lack thereof) are the end results of what we eat. Understanding how to choose and balance daily food is essential, if we are to be radiant and vital.

Yin and Yang

Yin and yang represent the two most fundamental concepts in any natural healing art. Rooted in an ancient understanding of nature, these concepts are used to describe natural phenomena in ways that are universally comprehensible. These two simple words sum up the foundation of the laws of nature.

The world in which we live is composed of an endless interplay of opposing forces, changing physical matter to energy and back again, in a continuing cycle of construction and destruction, expansion and contraction. The interaction of these two forces, termed *yin* and *yang* by Asian healers, creates an unending pattern of action and rest, which is evident in every aspect of nature.

Yin is a word symbolic of energy movement that creates expansion, moving outward, changing from the physical to the nonphysical. *Yang* symbolizes energy that is constricting in nature, moving toward the center, contracting, changing from the nonphysical to the physical. While opposite by nature, these two forces are not separate and do not act independently of each other. They work interdependently, in constant interplay with each other, forming one energetic interaction, constantly changing from one to the other and back again, expanding and contracting, creating the pulse of life in all of nature.

This basic concept of yin and yang forms the foundation for much of Eastern philosophical thought. In this pattern of thought and deduction, all of nature is seen as part of a whole.

A basic principle of Eastern thought is that everything changes; everything in nature is in a constant state of flux. This constant change is the norm, even in those cases where we don't actually see or experience the pulse of nature. It is considered to be the natural progression of nature, as expansion becomes contraction, that energy changes. As winter becomes spring, the weather changes. As we move from youth to aged, our bodies change. The only thing that never changes is that everything changes.

Yin and yang exist in all things, with expansion and contraction existing in all things, complementing each other as they interact, opening, closing, constructing and deconstructing, but never independent of each other. Either yin or yang will dominate. Every organism, phenomenon, or system will seem expansive or contracted in its apparent character, while its opposite nature will be minimized or even dormant. For instance, rocks appear to be hard and water soft and fluid, but rocks can be ground into sandy powder and water frozen into hard ice.

Yin and yang are merely different words, then, to describe a simple and basic principle of physics that all matter is composed of ever-changing energy. If we reconnect with nature and its rhythms, yin and yang become not only two words in our vocabulary, but terms that add meaningful dimension to our understanding of nature and our own character. When we understand the vital rhythms that govern us, we can be fully and responsibly involved in the creation and maintenance of our health.

Yin and yang is a philosophy of balance, which can be applied to understanding our human nature. Radiant health and beauty arise from the harmonious blending of expansion (yin) and contraction (yang) in the human form. We recognize this blending and are moved by the result of what we see. Our perception of harmony begins with shape, size, thickness, color, texture, and symmetry. When these qualities are balanced and proportioned, we perceive beauty and derive aesthetic pleasure from the appearance.

The harmonious balance between yin and yang are very important in creating a glowing, beautiful form. Think, for example, how society perceives obesity, an overly expanded human form. Our aversion is not a personal slight against any individual but rather a discomfort created by extreme imbalance. The same holds true when we see an overly thin or contracted human form. In both cases, our discomfort lies in the observation of imbalance. In our view as humans, an aesthetically pleasing form is one that illustrates expansion and contraction in proportion to each other. Think about how we view ourselves. When we perceive ourselves as too heavy or too thin, we grow upset and return to happiness only when we feel that our form is, once again, balanced.

In a similar manner, wet and dry and light and dark play important roles in our perception of balance and radiant health. For example, if the skin and hair become too contracted and dry, our skin pulls tight and we appear drawn, usually with dull hair. If the skin and hair grow too expanded and wet, we experience flaccid, loose skin and oily, limp hair. Beautiful skin, in our perception, is uniform and firm, with a bit of supple plumpness, balanced yin and yang. The same holds for color. A flawless complexion is one that is uniform in color, without patches of light or dark, redness, or spots. The uniform color that we all strive for with layers of foundation can be achieved by balancing yin and yang internally.

These simple examples show how harmony in our appearance is strongly influenced by the balance of yin and yang in the body. So what is that balance? What are the ideal proportions of expansion and contraction? They are rarely balanced in equal proportion—one or the other dominates. To understand the balance for the human form, we must understand the influence of yin and yang on the earth, begin to see how these energies appear to us and how they affect us as organisms that live on the planet.

The earth receives a tremendous amount of energy from outside itself, from the sun, moon, and other planets, as well as stars and other celestial bodies. This energy spirals toward the center of the earth and creates a yang, or contracting effect, on it. How do we see this force? Called gravity, we feel it as we are held to the surface of the planet or observe objects fall from our hands to the ground.

At the same time, the earth is constantly rotating and with this powerful motion, energy is moved in the opposite direction, creating an expansive energy around the planet. The interaction between these two forces creates the earth as we know it, from mountains to valleys, to plants that grow up toward the sun or drill into the soil, to streams to seas. It also creates plant and animal life. These two forces are not equal in their influence by any means. The force of the universe, the celestial (yang) influence, is far more powerful than that of the spinning of the globe (yin). It's obvious that things remain rooted to the surface of the earth and don't go flying off as the planet rotates. The balance of the two forces is about seven to one (as calculated in physics), with the force of the universe the stronger of the two. We see that same balance reflected in our human form as well. The length of the torso is seven times the height of the head. The length of the torso is seven times the width of the narrowest part of the waist. If the head is larger or smaller, or the waist is thicker than this average, the body strikes us as out of balance. It's clearly illustrated in how we react to gaining a bit of weight that expands our waistline. We begin to exercise to "shape up" because we have gotten "out of shape." We strive for the ideal balance.

Traditional Healing Arts

In my work and teaching, I employ many traditional healing concepts. All have their roots in traditional and Chinese medicine and will give you an overview of my view of life and health to help you better understand how to use this book.

Chinese medicine includes four methods of treatment: food, acupuncture, herbology, and physical manipulation. Contrary to popular myth, Chinese medicine was not developed or invented by any one particular individual, but rather grew and evolved out of the necessity to maintain good health. The ancient Chinese, just like us, struggled against disease and imbalance and in the process, came to discover the benefits of proper diet, medicinal herbs, and ways to physically move the body's internal energy to relieve symptoms or create vitality.

You may wonder why, with modern medicine, there's even a need for such ancient practices. It's because virtually any type of symptom can be effectively treated with traditional modalities. While I am not one to disparage modern Western medicine, there are distinctive differences between the modern idea of healing and more traditional views. Western medicine places its focus on treatment and relief of symptoms, while

Chinese medicine places its focus on the cause of said symptoms, which makes each modality useful to us in different situations. Modern medicine is without compare when symptoms are acute and the situation requires immediate results, as in an emergency, while Chinese medicine is most effective in cases of internal disease and chronic conditions. Modern medicine employs strong chemical drugs, which can produce extreme side effects in the body. Chinese medicine relies on natural herbs, food, and gentle manipulation of energy, which are less drastic, have long-lasting effects, and, when applied properly, produce very few, if any, side effects.

It is important to have as much information as possible about your medical condition. An accurate diagnosis—as you can get only from modern medicine—will serve you in making educated choices, whether conventional or alternative. We must learn, as patients and individuals, which approach to our condition is most appropriate so that we can best handle our situation.

Traditional Chinese medicine is based, for the most part, on a classic tome that was published in the third century, *The Yellow Emperor's Classics of Internal Medicine*. While many modern medical texts become obsolete as we learn more and more, the classic, basic principles that have guided traditional healing arts never change, because the laws of nature remain constant. What was appropriate for cleansing the liver, for example, in the third century, would be as effective today, since the liver does the same job in modern man that it did in ancient man. With that kind of ancient wisdom as the foundation and with the ever-growing understanding provided us by modern science, our understanding of the human species grows more complete. By basing our treatment of the human body on these principles of balance and harmony within nature, we can move our body to places where its natural instincts will take over and allow healing.

Since this classic text was published, there have been many other books written that build upon the foundation laid by this work. As a result, our understanding of nature's laws, Chinese medicine, and other alternative modalities has moved to a place of solid, credible effectiveness in the treatment and maintenance of human health.

Who Are We?

In our modern view, diagnosis identifies disease by observing symptoms. Chinese medicine, on the other hand, can often see a disease in the making before any symptoms actually arise. The principal tool of the Asian approach to healing is physiognomy, the art of judging a person from their facial features and line of the body. The basic premise of Chinese medicine is that each of us is a walking, talking history of our own development, encompassing our ancestry, culture, lifestyle, environment, and daily food choices. In our faces and bodies, we can observe everything about our family history, the health of our parents, the environment in which we grew, the food that nourished us during our development. All this and more is expressed in how we look, act, and feel. Everything about us, from the color of our skin to the tone of our voice to our posture is affected by our daily food choices, lifestyle, and environment.

Before visual diagnosis can be used effectively in our lives, there are aspects of humanity that must be understood. We must begin to grasp who we are and how we developed into the people that we see in the mirror each morning. We must begin at the beginning.

Our discovery of ourselves begins with discerning between constitution and condition. Our constitution is actually determined before birth, by familial characteristics, ancestry, the environment of our mother and of course, by her food choices during our embryonic development. The structure of our face, our bone structure, the shape of our hands and feet, the coloring of our hair and skin, the shape and color of our eyes, the shape of the head and body, sex, height, and tendency of weight are all determined by the conditions under which we develop in the womb. Our constitution is constant. We are unable to make ourselves taller or shorter, to change our brown eyes to blue or our fair skin to an olive complexion.

Our condition, on the other hand, is created on a daily basis. The texture of our skin and hair, the health of our nails, our weight, posture, stance, complexion, all these traits and more are determined by our daily choices, with food being one of the most influential.

OUR CONSTITUTION

According to classic Chinese medicine, people's physical and mental constitutions are formed under the following influences: hereditary factors from both our mother's and father's reproductive cells, the emotional and physical environment of our mother and her food choices during pregnancy.

In tandem with these factors, we must also take into consideration our parental and ancestral conditions, the date of our conception and birth, the place of our birth and childhood, the food choices of our mother during pregnancy, and family, social, and cultural conditions. Looking at each one, I'll show you how it relates to my own life, so you can see how it relates to your own.

Parental and ancestral conditions are the influences that affect us through generations, mostly in behavior. For example, families that are more physically oriented will most likely produce children that are similar to them in their behavior patterns. I come from a family of laborers. No matter what the profession, from attorney to homemaker to stone mason to carpenter, everyone worked hard, relishing that delicious feeling of exhaustion that comes at the end of a day of physical exertion. In turn, I feel my life is best when I am working hard, always busy and moving. While I exercise to remain fit, I would rather wash windows or mulch a garden for physical activity than take a turn on the stair machine. I find that "power yoga" serves my needs better than a more relaxed practice, for the same reason.

More sedentary families will, in general, produce offspring with the same tendencies. I have cousins who were raised in a more academically oriented family and they would rather pursue matters of study, have a debate, or read than sweat in a gym or a garden. One is not separate from the other. This is not to say that those who are physically oriented are more or less smart than the less active, or that academic people are slugs. These are tendencies, and if we observe closely, we can see them.

INFLUENCE OF THE DATES OF CONCEPTION AND BIRTH

The date and conception of our birth plays an important role in our inherent character, as there are many influences at play that create our constitutions. Studied in both Asian healing arts and western astrology, this is seen as one of the ways of determining destiny.

In physical terms, seasonal, atmospheric, electromagnetic vibrations, and celestial movements influence the physical and psychological conditions of people. We've all laughed at the full moon jokes of everyone being just a little crazy at that time of the month. But there is evidence that it's true. All of these conditions influence us energetically, creating different qualities in us as they change and shift.

In addition, eating patterns change with the seasons and months, oriented by the movement of the earth, sun, moon, and other planets, resulting in different blood quality at different times of the year. This difference in the quality of our blood is what creates different types of constitutions, even within the same family. It's very interesting to observe how dietary choices which change as the pregnancy progresses through various seasons, influence the constitutional qualities of the children. As weather changes from hot to cold and cold to hot, the mother's food and lifestyle choices change in accordance with the season. These climatic changes exert a strong influence on the child in the womb because of the mother's eating patterns. Thus, a child born in the spring will have a constitution that is opposite that of a child born in the autumn.

A person born in May is in the embryonic period from September, passing through autumn, winter and then born in the spring. During this time, the mother was most likely choosing foods that were heartier to compensate for the cold weather, such as stews, longer cooked foods, baked foods, maybe even more animal protein. This pregnancy will produce a very different child than the pregnancy that progresses from conception in March, culminating in birth in November. This child will have the influence of dietary patterns reflective of the spring and summer months, with lighter foods, more fruit, liquid, raw and fresh foods, and sweets. These children will have decidedly different constitutions, tendencies, and characters. In my own family, I am the only child born in the winter, in December, and I am quite different from my siblings in every way. Looks, temperament, character—you name it, we differ.

My husband and his brother, on the other hand, while three years apart in age, have birthdays just days apart in May and are like two peas in a pod, with similar temperaments, senses of humor, coloring, even mannerisms. So in my own family, I see evidence of the strong influence of the seasons when people are conceived and born. It may begin to explain for you, the sometimes seemingly great differences between siblings. Certainly, a family resemblance will remain, but our unique natures are born as a result of the many circumstances that surround our conception, gestation, and birth.

INFLUENCE OF CULTURE

The place of birth and childhood development also plays a role in determining our natures. In particular cultures, we see similarities. We use the clichéd phrases every day, oh, she looks Italian, or he doesn't look Jewish. These aren't ethnic slurs; they're just a way in which we recognize the similarities within a culture. These similarities come from the common factors that influence an entire people, from climate to eating patterns. And what we see, as cultures mixed and matched, relocated to various parts of the world, and began mating with different people, is a wide variety of people with as many characteristics as there are combinations.

Take hair color, for example. We commonly associate blond hair with Scandinavia, Ireland, Poland, areas of Russia, and the northern regions of Italy. Red hair is generally a characteristic of Ireland and some northern regions of Italy. Dark hair is associated with all Mediterranean regions, the Middle East, Asia, Africa, and the southern regions of the globe. So while you may no longer live in Sweden, your ancestry may still give you those traits. Most likely, though, you'll notice that the generations removed from the actual culture will look slightly different than their ancestors with deeper blond hair, slightly darker skin and eyes.

Red hair is said to be the result of a climate so cold and damp that it chills you to the bone. To stay warm, people consume more animal protein (high in iron and other minerals), along with the lack of sun, resulting in red hair and very pale skin that burns and freckles when exposed to sunlight. As people moved from the cultures that produce redheads, we see fewer and fewer of them—the real thing, anyway. Here in America, my flame-red hair has become something of a signature of my look. My father, who has always loved my hair and takes all the credit for it because of his Irish heritage, often laughs and says that if I were to return to our family's roots, my distinctive look would be commonplace, a dime a dozen, he likes to say.

As people mix and move around the globe, we notice that the most common hair color today is a compromise of dark and light, a mild brown color. As we have melded culturally and moved around the globe in search of our dreams, we have minimized the dramatic differences that culture and climate create, and grow enchanted by people that possess the strength of their cultural traits. We are fascinated by pale and lovely blondes, infatuated with the fiery flash of redheads, and fall in love with the drama of smoldering dark-haired beauty.

MOTHER'S FOOD CHOICES

Within each of these influences, the food choices made by the culture, family, father, and mother before pregnancy, and those made by the mother during pregnancy, play a large part. Even within a particular family, if the mother dramatically alters her eating patterns, she may produce a child that is quite different from the others, and even from the family. With today's family members eating differently and separately, rather than together, we see families that bear little resemblance to each other. You'll see a mother with children as different as night and day, with little in common in the way of looks and mannerisms. When families don't eat together, the quality of the blood that nourishes each person is different. The common bond that creates familial similarities starts with sharing the same kinds of foods, which create similar blood quality, which, in turn, creates a family that looks and acts like a unit, and can communicate with each other.

In my own family, my mother's cravings during her four pregnancies are the stuff of legend, and quite interesting to me in my current profession. With my brothers and sister, the story goes, Chinese take-out was the hands-down favorite. During my mother's pregnancy with me, and no one can explain the changes, she wanted only red-hot chile peppers and sausage. The result is that while a basic familial similarity exists between my siblings and me, I am different enough so that, as a child, my older brother had no trouble convincing me that I was adopted.

We can see here that our constitution is clearly influenced by many factors that take place before our actual birth. These influences create our inherent character, whether we will be tall, short, small or big boned, fair or dark, have blue, brown, gray or green eyes, with blond, red, black or brown hair that will be curly or straight, fine or thick. We will be born with a square, round or oval face, wide or close-set eyes, small or large nose, and long or short fingers.

Our constitution is only the beginning of who we are, however. Our basic body, face, and coloring are determined by the influences of our birth, culture, and health of our parents. It is our everyday choices that create *us* and determine the quality of our health, vitality, and appearance.

OUR CONDITION

It's here that we get to make some choices and actually determine the kind of person we are in the world. We do get to decide what we want to be when we grow up. We determine whether we're patient and kind or short-tempered. We decide if we're focused and clear or whether we muddle through the day. We choose whether we have strength and vitality or drag ourselves along, chronically exhausted. We determine if we live plagued by bad hair and skin, poor posture, concerns about weight or whether we, generally, are the best we can hope to be.

We create who we are and our appearance by the choices we make. One of my favorite hobbies is to observe people, listen to what they say, and connect the dots. Another favorite hobby is seeing films, so I have taken to using film stars as my examples for the study of diagnosis. Take Marlon Brando, for instance, whom I adore. So beautiful when he was young, smoldering on the screen, with strength, sexuality, and emotion, he has since grown less appealing, with a sluggish appearance. But if you observe him in old movies, even in his prime, you can see his tendency toward weight gain. There are appearances of excess even in his youthful face and body.

Now look at Tom Cruise, another favorite of mine. As a young actor, he had a youthful baby face, sweet, but lacking character and definition. As the years have gone by and he has grown into himself, his daily life choices, from a healthy diet to diligence in exercise to a maturing of personality, have created a beautiful specimen of what a human can be. His chiseled features, perfect skin, clear eyes, lustrous hair, and lean, fit body are a testament to his healthy life choices.

While we are not all Tom Cruise (he was very lucky with genetics), we all have the capability to be our absolute best, and to be less is to fly in the face of what it is to be human. Each of these beautiful men that I used as examples has made choices that have created the people that they are, as do we all. When we compromise our health and well-being, we squander the gift that is our life.

I am not saying that we must strive toward the impossible goal of perfection and that every woman is meant to be a size four and every man should look like a "GI Joe" doll. However, our daily life choices create the people we are and by making choices natural and appropriate to humans and with a bit of effort, we can be the very best that it is our inherent character to be. By doing that, we create health and vitality. With that comes a natural radiance that gives us that enviable glow that we strive for with artificial cosmetics. We can create natural beauty from within, and all with the choices we make every day.

Beauty Within Food

Food choices are the primary way in which we maintain the balance of yin and yang in the body and keep our physical condition and appearance in the greatest harmony with nature. We can begin to understand the power of food's effect on us, if we can begin to understand the classification of foods from yin to yang and how various foods will affect our overall appearance, as it affects our internal health.

In the broadest terms, for purposes of introduction to the concept, let's begin to classify foods from yin to yang in general terms.

In general, meat, poultry, eggs, dairy foods, seafood, fish, and other animal foods are considered to have more contracting, constricting, or tightening effects on the body and so are classified as having a more yang effect on us. Rich in hemoglobin, sodium and other contracting minerals, saturated fats, and heavy, dense proteins, these foods are very difficult for the body to digest, making it work hard and inefficiently to assimilate the nutrients. This added stress on the body causes it to contract, producing a yang condition.

On the other hand, foods from plant sources produce a more relaxing, even cooling effect in the body. Rich in chlorophyll and potassium, as well as other more expanded minerals, the fats and oils in plant food are lighter, less dense, and unsaturated. These kinds of foods provide us with fuel that burns more efficiently and allows energy to flow freely through the body, with no blockages to stagnate, which can cause everything from sluggish energy to dull skin and hair. Overall, when foods produce a more relaxed condition, they are said to be of a more yin nature and create a more yin condition in us.

A great deal of variation exists in classifying foods in terms of yin and yang energies. Some animal foods are more contracting than others, while even among vegetables, some are more expansive and others more tightening. For example, slow or inactive animals will yield a more expansive meat product for consumption. For example, octopuses slowly float through the water and are, therefore, more yin than shrimp, which dart about the sea. On the other hand, fish and seafood, in general, by their cold-blooded nature and water environment are more yin or expansive than land-bound animals, who are more evolved, move about more and are warm-blooded. These animals will have a more contracting effect in the body, with eggs as the most contracted form of animal food available. Eggs are the compacted, condensed energy of the entire animal, encased in a hard shell. This type of concentrated protein and energy will cause a great deal of stress in the body as it attempts to assimilate, resulting in constricted, tight organs, whose functions will be inhibited.

In the vegetable kingdom, the same natural laws hold true, with many factors impacting the overall nature of plants. For instance, climate plays an important role in the character of any given vegetable or fruit. When the climate is colder, plants create balance by becoming smaller and more compact, with less moisture and so are considered more yang or contracted. When the weather warms, plants respond by becoming more yin or expanded and moist to balance the warmth. For example, oranges and grapefruits, the result of hot, tropical weather, grow sweet and juicy to balance their environmental heat, while apples and pears, while still sweet, have far less juice and moisture. Carrots, which thrive in cold weather, drill into the soil, growing tight and compact, with little moisture, while lettuce, springs from the soil, opens its leaves to the sun and holds incredible amounts of water in the veins of its leaves to balance the heat of summer. These fruits and vegetables will all affect us differently, with the tropical fruits cooling us and the tree fruits relaxing us, while carrots give us warmth and strength and lettuce gently cools our bodies in summer heat.

Within the plant kingdom, whole grains are considered the center, since they are the perfect fusion of seed and fruit in one organism. It is said that whole grains are also the perfect reflection of the balanced proportion of yang and yin energies on the earth (seven to one), which is reflected in the balance of carbohydrates to proteins to minerals, each being seven to one, making whole grains quite balancing for us as humans.

In addition, whole grains are composed of complex carbohydrates which are most nourishing to us. Complex or long-chain carbohydrates are gradually broken down and are absorbed more slowly. On the other hand, the simple carbohydrates found in sugar, fruit, and fruit juice are composed of simple sugars that lack the cohesive nature of complex carbohydrates. These carbohydrates, in the form of sugars, are absorbed rapidly into the bloodstream, producing chaotic fluctuation in our metabolism, and we all know how that can affect both our health and our looks.

There are many other factors that influence the energy of food and, ultimately, its effect on our health and vitality. Cooking and processing are especially important, as they can change the character of a food most dramatically. The use of fire, pressure, salt, and time causes food to become more contracted (yang). Lighter methods of cooking and processing, along with the addition of oil or water, will open the foods, creating a more expanded (yin) energy. In studying cooking and processing, we see that these complementary forces are used to rebalance or alter the energy of food. When understood and applied with knowledge, these processes help us to create the harmony we seek within our environment, as well as serve our needs and desires. For instance, to effectively digest meat, beans, grains, and even some vegetables, they must be cooked or cured in some way, to begin to break them down. Then they will create less stress in the body, making for efficient use of the nutrients.

In terms of our radiant glow, climate plays an important role in choosing and balancing food. When eating to look and feel our best, we want to remain in harmony with our surrounding environment. To do that, we must choose, for the most part, foods from our own, or similar, climate. If you live in the northeastern region of the United States, a four-season climate and choose to eat many foods from the tropical state of Florida, you'll find yourself growing uncomfortable in the erratic weather that is the signature of the northeast. Think about how many people from a four-season climate (most of the world) indulge in orange or grapefruit juice every morning, then consider how many people want to retire to warm climates, because the cold weather is so uncomfortable for them. Coincidence? I think not. In order to balance our bodies within our external environment, we must align our internal environment with it, so that we fit in and are not creating imbalance, which in turn makes us uncomfortable and unattractive, which, left unchecked, will lead to "dis-ease."

There is no such thing as perfect balance or perfect health or perfect beauty, but we want to stay as close to the center of that personal balance as possible. Understanding food and creating internal harmony allows us to walk the tightrope that is balance with a bit more confidence, with delicate swaying to the left and right. We stay on the rope with fewer close calls.

Yin and yang are opposite energies and therefore attract each other. Choosing foods that are closer to the center of balance creates a calmer polarity in the body. The energy within us is less extreme. Choosing foods that are extreme yin or extreme yang, however, will create an atmosphere of tension and stress in the body as it struggles to maintain some kind of equilibrium. If that kind of extreme energy continues in the body and becomes its normal state of being, it becomes quite difficult to maintain. We begin to tire and wear down, with our vitality fading and our natural glow growing dim. Imbalance in the body that is allowed to continue will result in symptomatic conditions of the hair, skin, nails, and overall appearance.

Foods like whole grains, beans, bean products, seasonal fruits, and vegetables all contain yin and yang elements, but are easily balanced within the body, because their energies are not extreme. On the other hand, foods like animal protein, sugar, eggs, alcohol, and dairy, will be extremely dominated by either yin or yang energy and will therefore need an extreme opposite energy to make balance. For instance, we balance steak with raw salad or sweet dessert. Balance is created, but of such an extreme nature, the body grows exhausted from the sheer effort of eating. Rather than maintaining a vital, well-toned, firm body, we will experience the extremes of tightness in the muscles and joints, along with loose, flaccid skin, swelling, and lack of defined character, not to mention that we'll always feel less than great.

As you can begin to see, food has a direct effect on how we look. Eating well will create the foundation upon which we can build our vitality, which will show itself as natural, radiant health, and an enviable glow. Diet and lifestyle influence our appearance as they affect our health and vitality. Our skin, nails, and hair reflect the effect that our life choices are having on our overall well-being. Eating and living well will not only maintain, but can restore our body to optimum health and our appearance to natural radiance.

Balancing yin and yang in our lives, through our choices, is important for natural beauty and health. Yin and yang are invaluable in helping us to stay close to balance and avoid the extremes in life that can diminish our glowing vitality. Understanding the simple principles behind yin and yang can be invaluable in helping us to make the appropriate adjustments we need to be our best.

Finally, yin and yang help to clear up the mystery of the connection of body and mind, our physical and thinking selves. How we see ourselves is of the utmost importance in maintaining our health, and our radiant glow. Without a positive self-image, we will be less likely to make the effort needed to be our best. Begin by cultivating a peaceful mind and a positive outlook, in which you see yourself radiant with health. With this in mind, you will naturally seek to manifest that image by making daily choices that support your health and nourish your naturally beautiful self. Knowing that there is no perfection in beauty, accentuate the best in your appearance and see yourself as the naturally radiant, healthy being that you are. As you think, so you are. Living in harmony with nature, you will begin to radiate a deep, spiritual beauty that will light every part of your being and life. You will discover that your radiant glow comes from within and never fades but grows warmer with each passing year.

The Glowing
Face of Radiance

Looking in the mirror each morning can be . . . interesting at best. For some of us, it's downright terrifying. What face will we see today? What new sign of aging will have marched across our faces as we innocently slept? Will we be puffy-eyed or will we see dark rings under our weary bloodshot eyes? Are we pale and listless? Pimples? Blotches? Will we see more dreaded wrinkles? And then there are the bad hair days, which for many, are more the norm than the good ones.

It doesn't have to be that way. I remember watching a public television special on women's phases of aging. It interested me, because, well, I'm a woman and women tend to think a lot about aging. I was turning forty. I wasn't feeling particularly stressed about it, but maybe I was missing something. The information in the special was horrifying. It began with women in their twenties and talked about the prime of womanhood. The discussion moved to women's bodies in their thirties and the beginning of their decline. As they described what to expect, I was so depressed, I briefly considered ordering a walker. And then they reached women in their forties. I listened to the ways in which my body was about to degenerate in the next decade and grew intrigued, rather than upset. As I listened to predictions of hairs sprouting from my chin and the hair on my head thinning and everything, in general, beginning to point toward Venezuela, I realized that I hadn't even experienced the decline predicted in my thirties. What was up?

As usual, I reflected according to the principles by which I live my life. I realized that the predictions being made weren't so out of line. Considering the ways in which we overtax our bodies, how can we age in any other way than predicted? Our food choices are responsible for so much of our well-being and vitality, which is reflected in our posture, carriage, hair, and skin condition.

Now I am not so foolish or arrogant as to say that food is the only determining factor in our appearance. Food, however, is the foundation we build upon. Without superior quality, fresh food, the body grows tired and weak far more easily than if we were to make choices that serve to create optimal organ function. And the way in which the body functions, directly determines our day-to-day appearance. We *can* wake up, splash water on our face, run a hand through our hair and know we look our glowing best. It doesn't have to involve a major renovation every morning.

So how does it work? How do we apply esoteric information about yin and yang and energy to the practical living of our lives? We must re-establish a relationship with nature and begin to understand our deeply rooted connection with the earth. Strengthening that link creates an undeniable bond that will, instinctively, prevent us from making too many inappropriate choices that can result in the premature decline of our appearance.

With food choices as the foundation of your natural radiance, it is essential to discuss the impact of food's energy on our health and well-being. In order to understand what we are looking at when we examine our health by observing our faces, we must understand how food impacts us internally, since it will be reflected externally.

Food to Glow With

There are two inherent differences between the typical modern diet and a more holistic approach to eating. It seems that the focus of modern eating is weight loss, while a holistic pattern of choosing foods is based on understanding how food works to create the people that we are. By understanding the energy of food, we can choose wisely for whatever it is that we desire, from achieving our ideal weight to creating perfect skin and lustrous hair to supporting our bodies in the struggle to regain health, when a condition of illness arises.

I think the second difference is much more significant. In the modern approach to eating, foods are considered for their protein, calories, carbohydrates, fat, vitamins, and other nutrients. A holistic approach to eating, on the other hand, considers foods for their energies, movements, textures, and flavors, as well as nutritive value, and how all of these factors combine to create the character of food and the resulting effect of food on our body's vitality. Instead of dissecting food into its smallest molecules in an attempt to understand it, my view of food is reflected in how it affects me. When I feel cold, I like to eat foods that warm me; if I feel hot, I'll choose food that will cool my body. In both cases, I can choose foods to make me more comfortable. If I feel the muscles in my calves tighten from too much exercise or work, I can choose foods that will relax the tension gripping my legs. If my stomach feels weak, I can choose appropriately to help my tummy regain its strength. When I am chilled, I can eat ginger to drive warmth into my belly, and if I am uncomfortably warm, I can eat chile peppers to help my body disperse some of the heat held inside. Should I feel heavy or put on weight, I can choose foods that will aid me in releasing that excess and restoring my own balance.

Modern nutrition can give us all the information we need on what's *in* our food. We can look at a red chile pepper and discuss the vitamins A and C and potassium and we can read about the protein in tofu. In my view, however, none of this tells me what the experience of the food will be for me. It doesn't tell me that the chile pepper can help my body to release heat or that the tofu will help to relax muscle tension in my shoulders.

There are aspects of a holistic approach to eating that are essential to understanding food when you begin the study of self-diagnosis. They are the five flavors, the five energies, and the movement of food in the body and how it affects our internal environment.

THE FIVE FLAVORS OF FOOD

There are five tastes in food: sweet, pungent (spicy), salty, sour, and bitter. Each of these distinct flavors will affect us in different ways.

The flavors of foods are important in whole-foods cuisine, because each of the different flavors has its respective effect on specific organs or systems. This is especially important to us as we try to choose foods to maintain our natural radiant glow. Sweet foods act on the spleen, pancreas, and stomach; pungent foods on the lungs and large intestine; salty foods on the kidneys, bladder, and reproductive system; sour foods on the liver, gallbladder, and nervous system; and bitter foods on the heart, small intestine, and circulatory system.

These food flavors have been found, by centuries of experience, to have specific effects on specific organ systems, and by understanding these reactions to taste, we can manipulate our diet to achieve our goals. In general, the affects of the five flavors work in the body in the following ways: Sweet taste can slow acute symptoms and neutralize the toxic affects of other foods in the body. Pungent foods can work to induce perspiration and promote circulation. Salty foods can aid the body in softening the hardness of muscles, glands, and other tissue. Sour foods use their astringent nature to obstruct excessive movement and stem the loss of energy. Bitter foods help to reduce body heat and dry up excess fluid in tissue and organs. Utilizing the flavors of food with understanding, gives us the power to create a pattern of eating that satisfies our taste as well as nourishes our organs to function at *their* best, leaving us looking *our* best.

FOODS CLASSIFIED BY THE FIVE TASTES

Sweet Taste

Grains	Pumpkin	Honeydew melon
Millet	Rutabaga	Raisins
	Winter squash	
Beans		Sweet apples
Chickpeas		
		Sweet cherries
Vegetables	**Fruit**	
Green cabbage	Cantaloupe	Sweet grapes
Parsnip	Currants	Tangerines

Sweet Taste (Continued)

Sweeteners
Barley malt
Brown rice syrup

Nuts
Almonds
Pecans

Pungent Taste

Grains
Brown rice
Mochi
Sweet brown rice

Beans
Soybeans
Tofu
Tempeh
White beans

Vegetables
Bok choy
Carrots
Cauliflower
Celery
Chinese cabbage
Cucumbers
Daikon
Ginger
Leeks
Lotus root

Onions
Shallots
Turnips
Watercress

Fruit
Apricots
Peaches
Pears

Nuts
Walnuts

Salty Taste

Grain
Kasha

Beans
Adzuki
Black soybeans
Black turtle
Kidney
Pinto

Vegetables
Burdock
Radicchio

Red cabbage
Sea vegetables
Shiitake mushrooms
  and other
  mushrooms
Water chestnuts

Fruit
Blackberries
Blueberries
Chestnuts

Cranberries
Sour grapes
Watermelon

Condiments
Miso
Sea salt
Soy sauce
Tamari
Umeboshi plums
Umeboshi vinegar

Sour Taste

Grains
Barley
Oats
Rye
Wheat

Beans/Legumes
Black-eyed peas
Green lentils
Peanuts
Split peas

Vegetables
Alfalfa sprouts
Artichoke
Broccoli
Green beans
Green peas
Lettuce
Parsley
Summer squash

Fruit
Granny Smith apples
Lemons

Limes
Plums
Pomegranates

Oils
All

Pickles
Olives
Sauerkraut
Sour pickles

Bitter Taste

Grains
Amaranth
Corn
Quinoa

Beans
Red lentils

Vegetables
Arugula
Asparagus

Belgian endive
Broccoli rabe
Brussels sprouts
Chile peppers
Chives
Collard greens
Dandelion greens
Kale
Mustard greens
Red bell peppers

Scallions
Snow peas

Fruit
Raspberries
Strawberries
Oranges
Tomatoes

Nuts/Seeds
Sesame seeds
Sunflower seeds

Extreme Foods

Bell peppers
Chocolate
Coffee

Eggplant
Potatoes
Sugar

Tropical fruits and
vegetables

THE FIVE ENERGIES OF FOOD

The energies of foods are simply descriptions of how foods will act in the body and our resulting sensations, hot, cold, warm, cool, or neutral.

To see how these energies are useful to us, we must understand that each adjective—warm, cool, hot, cold, or neutral, does not necessarily refer to the actual food, but to its effect in the body. For example, tea is considered to have a cold energy, but when we drink it, it is physically hot. Once in the body, however, its heat dissipates quickly, cooling the body, making it the perfect summer refresher. If you choose to eat a red chile pepper, it may feel cool to the touch (if not to the mouth), but once in the body, its natural heat is released and we feel its warmth build inside us. So the understanding of the energies of foods has to focus on what foods do in the body. Do they generate heat, chill us, or serve to bring things into balance with their neutral nature?

The importance of understanding the energetic effect of foods in our bodies is directly related to our good health and resulting radiant glow. For example, if you suffer from skin problems that worsen in the heat, eating foods that warm you will make the symptoms more acute, while choosing cooling foods will alleviate the severity of the symptoms, as they draw energy away from the problem. If your skin grows dry in cold weather, then choosing foods that chill the body will only make matters worse, while warming foods will soothe and nourish your parched skin. Choosing foods with neutral energy can help to restore the body to balance in a gentle manner.

The effect of food energies is individual, so we need to understand ourselves a bit before we can utilize this information to our best advantage. When I am teaching or lecturing, I am often asked questions like: Is tea good? Is coffee bad? Is ice good? Is meat bad? These are not bad questions, simply the wrong ones. The questions should be framed to ask: Is tea good for me? Then we can examine our personal constitution and tendencies and make a choice. One man's food is another man's poison.

FOODS CLASSIFIED BY THE FIVE ENERGIES

Cooling Energy

Apples

Arugula

Barley

Collard greens

Cucumbers

Daikon

Dandelion

Kale

Lettuce

Marjoram

Mung beans

Mushrooms (button)

Pears

Peppermint

Pineapples

Radishes

Strawberries

Tofu

Watercress

Wheat

Cold Energy

Bamboo shoots

Bananas

Bay leaf

Grapefruit

Salt

Sea Vegetables

Sugar

Tomatoes

Watermelons

Neutral Energy

Apricots

Azuki beans

Black sesame seeds

Brown rice

Cabbage

Carrots

Chinese cabbage

Celery

Corn

Daikon tops

Figs

Grapes

Green beans

Kidney beans

Kohlrabi

Licorice

Lotus seeds

Olives

Parsnips

Plums

Potatoes

Pumpkin

Radish leaves

Shiitake mushrooms

Sunflower seeds

Sweet potatoes

Umeboshi plums

Yellow and black
   soybeans

Warming Energy

Asparagus

Basil

Buckwheat

Burdock

Caraway

Chestnuts

Chives

Cinnamon sticks

Cloves

Coffee

Coriander

Fennel

Garlic

Ginger (fresh)

Ginseng

Leeks

Millet

Mustard greens

Peaches

Quinoa

Raspberry

Rosemary

Scallions

Vinegar (all)

Walnuts

Wine

Hot Energy

Black pepper

Cinnamon bark

Chile peppers

Dried ginger powder

Green bell peppers

Red bell peppers

Soybean oil

White pepper

Depending on their character, foods will move inward, outward, rise in the body, or sink, affecting us in decidedly different ways. I think of the body as divided into four regions: interior, exterior, above the waist, and below the waist, all connected, but with different needs and tendencies.

Foods that move outward impact us by driving energy to our surface, the skin. Foods with this character will cause the skin to react, inducing perspiration and helping to reduce fever. These foods may also aid in the discharge of excess, stagnant energy, again, by pushing it outward. These foods are strong and will have a tremendous effect on us.

Foods with inward movement can aid the body in contracting or tightening and can be quite effective in strengthening flaccid, loose skin and organs. These foods can aid in the relief of swelling in the torso or limbs. They can be used to strengthen digestion and reduce swelling in the abdomen as they work to pull energy to our center, helping us to feel stronger and centered.

Foods that rise in the body can help us to feel lighter and refreshed, as they move energy from deep in the body, up and out. These foods can be especially helpful in relieving lethargy and heaviness in the lower body. If energy is moving up and out, it is unlikely that we will feel heavy and lazy. Foods of this nature can aid in weight loss and gracefulness.

Foods that sink or move downward in the body can help us to feel more grounded and strong. These foods give us strength of character and the ability to feel powerful. They are also quite effective when dealing with nervous energy, anxiety, and lack of focus. By drawing the energy of the food deep into the body, we feel very nourished, focused, calm, and sure of our strength. Foods of this nature can help to strengthen flaccid muscles and improve our sense of balance, great for athletes or even weekend warriors.

The movements of foods are related to the flavors and energies of foods, and when applied to cooking, can serve us as we choose. Generally speaking, foods that are sweet or pungent will be warming and will tend to move inward or downward in the body. Foods with salty flavor can be warming or cooling, but will tend to move downward. Foods with sour taste tend to rise and have a cooling energy. Bitter-flavored foods tend to move outward and can have a cool or hot energy.

Foods can also be classified by their season. Foods with rising energy are associated with spring; foods with outward movement are enlivened by summer; foods that move downward are associated with autumn; and foods with inward-moving energy are enlivened by winter. With this in mind, seasonal food choices become even more important to the maintenance of our natural, radiant glow.

We can use all this information to create our health and vitality. For instance, if you are experiencing symptoms associated with weakness, energy leaving the body, generally a cold condition, which would be the result of excessive outward movement, you can get relief and draw strength by using warming foods that move energy inward and downward in the body. Balancing the various energies, flavors, and movement tendencies in foods are the key to glowing health, with achieving balance as the goal. Excesses in any of the energies, flavors, and movements will continue to create conditions of discomfort, rather than harmonious health.

FOODS CLASSIFIED BY MOVEMENT PATTERNS

Upward Movement

Apricots
Arugula
Black sesame seeds
Barley
Celery
Chinese cabbage
Chives
Collard greens
Dandelion
Figs
Grapes
Kale
Kohlrabi
Leeks
Lemons
Lettuce
Olives
Peanuts
Plums
Saffron
Scallions
Shiitake mushrooms
Sunflower kernels
Tempeh

Outward Movement

Black pepper
Chile peppers
Cinnamon bark
Coffee
Dried ginger
Green bell peppers
Red bell peppers
White pepper
White sugar

Downward Movement

Apples
Adzuki beans
Bananas
Black soybeans
Brown rice
Daikon
Carrots
Kidney beans
Mung beans
Parsnips
Peaches
Pears
Pumpkins
Strawberries
Sweet potatoes
Tofu
Winter squash

Inward Movement

Bay leaf
Burdock
Ginger (fresh)
Salt
Sea vegetables

So what does all of this have to do with putting our best face forward each day? As you'll see, the association between our internal environment and our outward appearance is quite clear. Just as foods have their specific inherent characters, their effect on our organs can be just as specific. In the Asian healing arts, the impact of food on our organs was discovered through treatment methods. If a certain food was found to be helpful in the relief of disease, then that food was considered good for specific action in that organ. After observing many instances of response of organs to food, certain associations were made between foods and their impact on the health of certain organs (see pages 66–73).

The Glowing Connection

As we observe ourselves and others, we must establish the link between our constitution and condition (see pages 10–15) in order to see our health.

During fetal development, our navel functioned as the center of our being, the center of our structure. As we developed internally, we developed externally (balancing yin and yang), and so as organs developed inside the body, our face was developing as an external balance. The result is that we can observe our internal health by observing our faces and discerning between constitution and condition. With this kind of understanding of our bodies, we can see our health. Along with this ability to observe, we also have the ability to act on what we see, because we have developed an understanding of the effects of food on organ health and can become proactive in affecting change.

After birth, the center of the body shifts to the mouth and neck region. From here, upper and lower extensions of the body develop, with the head as the upper sphere and body as the lower sphere. As a result, they correlate very well during development. According to this ancient principle, specific areas of the face reflect the condition and function of each organ of the body (see drawing below). We "grow into" our faces, as we mature and develop internally.

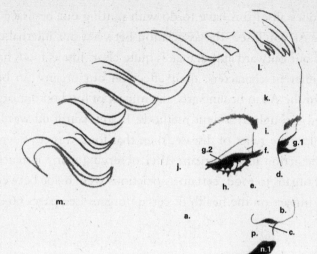

FACIAL AREAS AND THEIR CORRESPONDING ORGANS

a. Lungs

b. Heart

c. Bronchi (connecting the lungs)

d. Stomach

e. Liver

f. Pancreas

g. Kidneys, ovaries, testicles

  g-1. Spleen, pancreas

  g-2. Liver, gallbladder

h. Kidneys

i. Liver

j. Spleen

k. Small intestines; peripheral area of forehead, large intestines

l. Bladder

m. Kidneys

n. Digestive system

  n-1. Stomach

  n-2. Small intestines

  n-3. Large intestines

o. Duodenum

p. Reproductive organs

q. Reproductive organs

r. Kidneys

So what does all this mean to us? What makes a glowingly healthy face? Once you know where to look to find the health of various organs, it's important to know what you are looking at, how to see imbalance, what the imbalance is, and, most important, how to shift the imbalance back to the center, so that you look your best. Let's take it from the top. Grab a mirror and let's take a look.

First, no one has a perfectly symmetrical face. One side will vary slightly from the other, one eye may be a bit larger, one nostril shaped slightly differently, the nose may bend either left or right. These dissimilarities are part of our constitution and are caused by differences in the health and strength of our parents during conception and pregnancy, which create different influences in our development. In classic Asian healing, it is said that the health of the father influences the left side of the body and the mother influences the right side, both inside and out.

On the face, and internally, we can see who was constitutionally more influential quite easily. For example, if the left eye is more defined and strong, your father was stronger than your mother during your conception. Wherever you see specific, defined traits, you can determine the constitutional strengths of your parents, depending on which side shows more strength and definition. You can take this further. For example, you have a more defined left eye, but in examining your life, most of your injuries, accidents, and disorders have occurred on the left side. That indicates that while your father was quite a strong influence at the time of conception, your mother was a stronger influence during pregnancy and gave you greater strength on the right side, overpowering your father's influence. It is said in Asian healing, for instance, that most people are right-handed because our mothers' influence is stronger, since we spend the nine months after conception in her womb.

People who appear to be symmetrical are people whose parents maintained similar strengths and health from conception to birth. Familial influences run much deeper than whether we got our mother's eyes or our father's chin.

The Forehead
More than just the area of our head that we slap in frustration, the forehead is said to reflect the condition and function of the intestines. It is an indication of our overall mental and physical condition. For pur-

poses of Asian healing, the forehead can be divided into four sections, upper forehead, middle forehead, lower forehead, and temples.

Upper Forehead

This region of the forehead, immediately below the hairline, shows the function of the circulatory and excretory systems, heart, kidneys, and bladder. When this area is well-developed, with smooth, clear skin, these organs are functioning at their best. Any abnormal changes that occur in color or texture are indicative of imbalance in these organ systems.

Red skin color indicates that the circulatory system is overworked and aggravated, due to the excessive consumption of liquid, in particular, fruit juices, alcohol, coffee, and other stimulating beverages. The red color is often accompanied by a faster pulse, frequent fevers or flushes, and indigestion.

White skin color or patches of white will appear with the excessive consumption of dairy fats. Often found coupled with tiny, silver "baby hairs," this condition is indicative of high levels of cholesterol and fatty acids in the bloodstream. A weakened heart can result if this condition is left unchanged.

Dark skin color or patches of darker skin are caused by the excessive consumption of simple sugar, including fruit and fruit juice, white flour products, honey, maple syrup, and other simple sugar products. Cysts and stones from accumulating fat around the kidneys as well as frequent bladder infections, are just two of the symptoms that often accompany this condition.

Yellow skin color or patches of yellow show the skin's attempt to discharge excess fat and protein from meat, poultry, eggs, and cheese. You may also find this discoloration in people who eat large amounts of fatty fish or who take fish oils as a supplement to their diet. This condition is often accompanied by dysfunction of the liver and gallbladder, with a high cholesterol level in the bloodstream.

Pimples on this area of the forehead are an attempt by the body to eliminate some kind of excess. Red pimples are from sugar; white pimples are from fats; yellowish pimples are from animal protein and cholesterol; dark pimples are from dense protein and fat together, like those found in meats.

A receding hairline, showing as a balding forehead, is caused by the excessive consumption of sweets, fruit, juices, and alcohol over a long period of time. This condition shows that the heart and circulatory system are overworked because the quality of the blood and lymph has been compromised and is thinner and weaker, thereby working the heart much harder in order to service the body's needs, weakening the hair follicles so that they can not hold the hair in place.

Middle Forehead

This area shows the health and function of the nervous system. When this area is clear and well developed, it is an indication of healthy nervous function. Any changes or disorders in this area are signs of nervous dysfunction.

Red skin color, which is due to the overconsumption of stimulants and soft drinks, is often accompanied by frequent nervousness, anxiety, oversensitivity, and emotional instability.

White skin color or white patches, caused by an excess of dairy foods in the diet, are often accompanied by dulled nervous response and cloudy mental activity.

Yellow skin color, caused by excessive amounts of eggs and poultry in the diet, are accompanied by a nervous response that is alert, but narrow and inflexible, unable to adapt well to change. A similar condition is often found in vegetarians who take in large amounts of carrot juice, indicating an overworked gallbladder. Balance is important in all areas of eating, even veggies.

Dark spots or freckles indicate the body's attempt to eliminate simple sugars, medications, and chemicals. A balanced diet can help to fade these spots.

Red pimples are the body's attempt to eliminate excessive consumption of white flour products and dairy foods.

Look at the lines across your forehead. When you raise your eyebrows, creases appear. When you relax your face they should disappear, regardless of age. Three horizontal lines across the middle forehead are normal; any more than that is an indication that we are consuming too much food, healthy or not. We used to develop these lines as we aged, after years of overeating. Now we see them in younger and younger people, as we eat more and more. At the same time, notice older people without craggy foreheads. They most likely came from leaner times and are not accustomed to consuming large quantities of food.

Lower Forehead

This area of the forehead represents the respiratory and digestive systems of the body, as well as being reflective of their condition. It is also said that sensor discrimination is reflected in this area of the forehead. When clear and well developed, this area shows efficient function of these two systems, with our mental energies being clear and focused. Any changes or disorders in this area are indicators that there are dysfunctions in the respiratory and digestive systems.

Red skin color shows that our digestive function is aggravated, with expansion in the stomach and intestines occurring, with the accumulation of fat and mucus around the organs. Caused by overeating of extreme foods, both animal fats and protein, as well as simple sugars, this condition is also indicative of inflammation in the respiratory system.

Dark skin color or patches of dark color indicate that metabolism in the respiratory and digestive systems are slowed as a result of excess animal protein in the diet, particularly meat, eggs, cured meats, and salt. This condition is often accompanied by shortness of breath and chronic constipation.

White skin color or white patches represent the body's attempt to eliminate accumulations of fat and protein around the lungs, stomach, and intestines, mainly due to excessive consumption of poultry, eggs, cheese, and milk. This condition can be accompanied by both loose bowels and constipation.

Red pimples indicate that the body needs to eliminate excesses of sugar, fruit, juices, and chemicals.

Green skin color is an indication of serious dysfunction of the respiratory and digestive systems. Caused by overeating, especially extreme foods such as meat, eggs, sugars, and fruits; this condition very likely indicates that cysts and possibly tumors are forming in the lungs, stomach and intestines.

Central Region of the Lower Forehead (between the eyebrows)

This area reflects the health and function of the liver and gallbladder. When clear and free of lines, hair, pimples, puffiness, or other disorders, we can be confident that our liver is happy and doing its job well. Abnormalities in this area of the forehead indicate that our liver needs our attention.

The most commonly seen disorder in this area are vertical lines between the brows. Seen more often than not in modern people, these little lines are indicative of fat and mucus accumulating in the liver, causing hardness and expansion of the organ. The longer and deeper the lines, the worse is the condition of the liver. Sometimes you see one line, sometimes many lines. The more lines, the harder the liver is. Small lines that come and go are indicative of the liver's response to fatty foods. Greasy take-out tonight can mean little lines between the brows tomorrow. The good news is that these tiny lines will often disappear by noon. However, should greasy take-out become a food group for you, these lines will deepen, lengthen, and not go away so easily, as the liver continues to overwork and harden. The liver is associated with impatience and anger in the Asian healing arts. People with these little lines tend towards short tempers and impatience; we appropriately call them "frown lines."

Puffiness in this area is indicative of excessive consumption of sweets, causing the liver to swell and grow flaccid. Usually accompanied by a yellowish pallor, this condition is often accompanied by feelings of self-pity.

Moving down ever so slightly to the top of the bridge of the nose, just below the area between the brows, we see the condition and health of the pancreas. If horizontal lines appear in this area, the pancreas is growing hard from overwork and is seriously in need of some vacation time. Caused by excessive consumption of shellfish, eggs, and on the other end of the spectrum, simple sugar and sweets, this condition is more commonly found today and can be an indication that there is serious pancreas trouble on the way. A diet change is in order here.

White or yellow patches in this area indicate that gallstones may be developing as fat continues to accumulate in the liver, causing it to swell and harden.

Pimples in this area of the forehead indicate that hard fat deposits are forming in the liver and stones in the gallbladder, both due to excessive consumption of animal protein, particularly meat and eggs.

If the skin in this area grows dry and flaky, your diet may be excessive in the consumption of fats, both animal and vegetable. Even good-quality oils can cause this condition, if eaten in excess. This condition can also indicate a lack of adequate vegetable consumption.

Temples

These areas of the forehead correspond to the health and function of the spleen, pancreas, liver, and gallbladder. Clear, smooth, and free of puffiness, the temples indicate smooth, efficient function of these excretory organs.

Green-colored vessels in the temples indicate that the lymph circulation is abnormal due to an overactive spleen and underactive gall bladder, both conditions caused by excessive consumption of fluids and simple sugar, alcohol, and stimulants.

Dark color on the temples indicates that the body is trying to eliminate excessive amounts of extreme foods from the body, including sugar, honey, maple syrup, chocolate, fruits, syrups, milk, and white flour, as well as salts, cured meats, and hard, dry foods. This skin conditions shows that the liver, spleen, and kidneys are sluggish, while the pancreas function grows erratic in response to excessive sugar in the diet.

Pimples or discoloration on the temples indicate the body's effort to eliminate excess from these organs, everything from sugar and meat to salt and refined flour products.

Overall, the forehead is indicative of our entire physical health. A clear, smooth forehead shows that our organ systems are functioning smoothly with various metabolisms in harmony.

Our Eyes and Eyebrows

Eyebrows

They say that the eyes are the windows to the soul, making the eyebrows the awnings. In the Asian healing arts, the eyes and eyebrows reveal a great deal about our constitutional and conditional health. Your eyes and eyebrows conceal nothing.

The eyebrows reflect the health and condition of the nervous, digestive, circulatory, and excretory systems. In other words, every organ system in the body is shown here. The eyebrows reveal how our constitution developed during our gestation, as well as revealing our condition on a day-to-day basis.

By looking at eyebrows, we can see the state of the mother's health during pregnancy. The inner portion of the brows reflect the first trimester, the middle of the brow, the second trimester, with the outer tips of the brows showing the final months of development. By examining the eyebrows, we can determine a lot about constitutional strengths and weaknesses.

The space between the eyebrows is created by the mother's eating habits, especially during the third month. A more narrow space is created when a woman chooses more animal protein, salt, or long-cooked vegetables, seasoned with lots of salt during pregnancy, while a wider space is the result of more fruit, sugars, raw foods, or tropical foods.

More narrow spaced brows show that, constitutionally, our more compact organs, the liver, pancreas, kidneys, and heart, will be our inherent weak spots and require more tender loving care during our life. Wider-spaced brows reflect inherent weakness in our more expansive organs, the lungs, intestines, bladder, and gallbladder.

The more narrow the space, it is said, the more strong-willed, determined, and stubborn the personality. A wider space between the brows creates a personality that is more easygoing, even to the point of indecisiveness.

The angle of the eyebrows is quite telling and very interesting. This aspect of the eyebrows shows mental and physical strength. Upward-slanting brows (going up at the outer tips) are formed by the excessive consumption of animal protein by the mother during pregnancy. These eyebrows reveal great physical strength but also strong aggression in the personality. These people are also prone to liver and heart trouble in life should they neglect their health.

Downward-slanting brows (pointing down at the outer tips) are the result of minimal animal protein in the mother's diet during pregnancy, with the majority of the diet coming from vegetable sources. This personality is more passive and gentle, with the kidneys and intestines needing more attention than other organs.

Peaked brows, looking almost pointed as they arch at the center, are created when the diet chosen by the mother during pregnancy was more erratic, bouncing from excesses of animal food to excesses of sugar and fruit. The personality associated with these brows is a person who is physically active, socially gentle, appearing quite strong but with periods of timidity. Usually, these people are quite physically active in their early lives but turn to spiritual practices later in life. In these people, the extremes in food choices can contribute to weakness in the spleen, liver, and kidneys throughout life.

Brows with a more balanced angle, beautifully arched and graceful, are created when a mother chooses a well-balanced diet throughout most of her pregnancy. These brows reflect an overall physical strength and mental and emotional stability.

The hair quality of the eyebrows is reflective of inherent vitality. The denser the brows, the more vitality, while the thinner the brows, the more delicate is the constitution. It is important to note that as we age, the brows usually begin to thin, especially if our health grows delicate. If we have been seriously ill during our life—even in youth and even if we recover fully—the brows may thin. Physical trauma or malnourishment may cause thinning of the brows. So it is important to know what a person's life has been like before diagnosing them at a cocktail party.

It is said that the length of the brows is indicative of the length of life. Longer brows, which indicate strong vitality, indicate longevity while shorter brows can point to a shorter life and more delicate constitution.

Hair growing between the brows is said to be caused by the excessive consumption of dairy food and fatty animal food by the mother during the first trimester of pregnancy. A personality with this tendency in the brows will be easily affected by the consumption of animal protein and fatty foods as their liver, pancreas, and spleen have more delicate natures.

Finally, it is said that eyebrows with breaks or irregular growth of hair indicate a tendency toward serious illness at some point during life. Note, of course, that all of our constitutional tendencies can be altered with healthy life choices. This self-knowledge gives us an edge on maintaining our health, understanding our inherent strengths and weaknesses, so we know where to focus our self-care.

Eyes

The eyes, those most hypnotic parts of the face, tell it all. When we are feeling well and at our best, the eyes are powerful, clear, sharp, alert, seductive, and soulful, revealing all about our moods and desires. When our health is in decline, we see it all too clearly in our eyes, as they lose their clarity, power, and strength.

The study of the eyes can be a lifelong passion. It seems the more that we look at the eyes, the more we learn about the miracle of humanity. Here, we will discuss how to see our day-to-day health and what the eyes reveal about both our constitution and our daily condition. Representing our entire physical and mental condition, the eyes are our most expressive tool, reflecting every change, trauma, imbalance, and balance in our nature. They reveal everything about us.

Eye Placement, Size, and Shape

Beginning with our constitution, there is the size, shape, and placement of the eyes to consider. Close-set eyes are created by the consumption of more animal protein by the mother during pregnancy and indicate a sharp intelligence and intense nature. Wide-set eyes are created by the mother consuming more expansive foods like fruit, sugars, raw foods, and salads and indicate a gentle, more passive character with a more poetic nature.

The angle of the eyes is quite interesting. Eyes that slant upward at the outside corners, as in Asian eyes, are said to be the result of a mother's diet rich in long-cooked and strongly salted foods, as in the typical Asian diet, which includes heavy amounts of salt, longer pickled foods, and long-cooked grains. The character associated with these eyes is said to be more intellectually oriented.

Eyes that slant downward at the outside corners are said to be created by the mother having a more relaxed diet with very little salt and a tendency toward very lightly cooked vegetables and more fruit. These eyes are said to reflect a more passive, peaceful, and accepting character.

Eyes with no strong slant in either direction reflect the mother having a diet that was more balanced during pregnancy, with both strong cooking and light, fresh foods in balance. These eyes reflect a balanced nature, with both strength and peacefulness present.

The size of the eyes indicates basic characteristics in our personality. Smaller eyes, caused by the mother's consumption of well-cooked foods, both animal and vegetable, indicate a determined, self-confident character with strong vitality and endurance. Larger eyes, caused by the mother's consumption of lightly cooked foods, more sweets and juices, indicate a more delicate and gentle nature, with a tendency toward more creative thinking.

Eyelashes

Longer eyelashes are caused by the mother's intake of more sweets and fruits during pregnancy and indicate a gentle, romantic personality, while shorter lashes are caused by a diet rich in well-cooked animal and vegetable foods and is said to indicate a more pragmatic nature.

Eyeball

Looking at the eyeball itself, much is revealed about our health. Part of the nervous system, the eyeballs indicate a great deal about our overall health.

Iris and Pupils: The iris, which differs in color based on ancestry, constitution, and environmental conditions of the mother during pregnancy, is reflective of our various cultures and traditions. A lighter iris, blue, green, or light gray, indicates a person with ancestry from more northern parts of the world, where there is less cumulative sunlight. A light- or medium-brown iris, the two most common iris colors, is created in a temperate, four-season climate, where we experience both sun and clouds. Dark-brown and nearly black iris colors are created in sunny, tropical environments.

Using the iris, a method of diagnosis known as iridology was developed by Dr. Bernard Jensen and is a life-long study. The basis of iris diagnosis is that each spot, dot, line, and color means something in the body. Divided into many sections, a general view is that the upper part of the body, neck, face, and brain are reflected in the upper portion of the iris; the sides reflect the middle body, the thorax and lungs; the lower portion of the iris reflects the lower body, from the abdomen to the pelvis. Any abnormality in the iris reflects an imbalance in a particular organ or system. Accurate and always fascinating, iridology is a tried-and-true method of diagnosis used in many natural healing modalities.

The pupils of the eyes clearly reflect the health and function of the autonomic nervous system. Responding to the brightness or dimness of the surrounding environment, the pupils allow the light we need into the eyes. The speed of the response to changes in light indicates the alertness of the autonomic nerves.

Finally, the iris should be clearly defined around its perimeter; a cloud around the rim of the iris indicates that there is a high level of cholesterol and fat accumulating in the bloodstream.

Whites of the Eyes: The whites of the eyes reveal even more about us. Representing, as the iris does, various organ systems of the body, the whites of the eyes are a bit easier to read and diagnose. The whites of the eyes are divided in a similar manner to the iris.

The upper part of the whites of the eyes reflect the health and function of the upper body, including the brain, face, neck, chest, lungs, heart, and upper spine. The middle whites reflect the health of the middle of the body, including the stomach, duodenum, spleen, pancreas, liver, gallbladder, kidneys, and midspine. The lower whites of the eyes show the health of the lower body, including the small and large intestines, bladder, reproductive organs, buttocks, and lower spine.

The whites of the eyes should be just that, white. Any discoloration, marks, lines, spots, or other changes to them indicate that imbalances exist in the body.

A yellow color, particularly around the peripheral areas of the white indicates an accumulation of fat in the liver and gallbladder. In the case of yellowing, the fat is generally from vegetable oils or fish. A blue color, on the other hand, indicates an accumulation of harder fats in the liver and gallbladder, generally from more dense animal protein, like meat, eggs, and poultry.

Gray or dark patches, most often seen in the middle regions of the whites, indicate sluggish function in the organs and glands, including disorders in lymphatic function.

A translucent, pale color, like a cloud over the whites, indicates advanced accumulation of congestion and fat, which is progressing toward the formation of cysts in the body. Lymph and hormonal imbalances are often present as well.

Overall red coloring in the whites is caused by expanded capillaries and indicates irregularities in the circulatory and respiratory functions. Caused by excessive consumption of simple sugar, alcohol, caffeine, and other stimulants, this condition shows that the circulatory and respiratory systems are overworked and aggravated.

A straight red line in the whites of the eyes is somewhat rare but significant. It indicates abnormal malformation of muscle, tissue, or blood vessels. This condition is caused by a physical trauma like an accident or surgery and shows up in the whites in the corresponding area of the damaged tissue.

Red spots and broken veins that accumulate in the whites of the eyes indicate circulatory stagnation in various organs, glands, and muscles of the corresponding organs.

If dark spots appear here and there in the whites, it is an indication of a more serious accumulation of fat in the body, possibly progressing toward the formation of cysts and even tumors. This is a condition that requires our attention; ignoring it can lead to more serious health concerns.

Examining the insides of the upper and lower eyelids can be very telling. When we are balanced and healthy, the insides of the lids will be smooth and pink. When an imbalance occurs in the body, certain changes can occur.

If the interior eyelid color is more red than pink, this indicates an expansion of blood vessels caused by excessive consumption of simple sugar, sweets, soft drinks, caffeine, and other stimulants or chemicals. This condition can indicate difficulties with reproductive functions.

If the coloring turns red with a yellowish cast, then fat is hardening and accumulating around the heart, liver, and kidneys, and the blood vessels are expanding.

Very pale pink or white color is a clear indication of anemia and can be caused by excessive consumption of either (or both) salt or simple sugar, sweets, and artificial chemicals.

Tiny pimples on the insides of the lids show the body's attempt to eliminate excessive saturated fat from meat, eggs, poultry, dairy foods, and even fish.

Finally, if the eyes appear to be red-rimmed around the perimeter of the eyelids, as though a red line was drawn around them, but not in the whites or inside the lids, this indicates a condition of immune dysfunction. Our natural defenses are weakening as the body continues to overwork to defend itself.

Skin Around the Eyes

We spend billions of dollars to preserve, revive, and refresh the delicate skin around the eyes. The color of the skin around the eyes varies according to our health and can change daily based on our lifestyle and diet choices. Clear, smooth skin around the eyes is a clear indicator that our physical and emotional health is balanced and harmonious. Color changes can occur in any area of skin around the eyes but is most dramatically seen in the skin just below the eyes.

Dark skin color under or around the eyes occurs when the kidneys and adrenal glands grow exhausted and can be caused by the excessive consumption of dense, dry, or salty foods as well as excessive strain from activity and stress. With this condition, the function of the kidneys grows stagnant and the organs themselves dry, and over time, if ignored, the individual will grow weak with constricting tightness in the lower back.

Reddish color anywhere on the upper eyelids or under the eyes is caused by simple sugar, excessive amounts of fruit, chemicals, medications, and stimulants and indicates that the heart and circulatory system are overworked and aggravated. Interestingly, this condition can come and go, often appearing when we are nervous or, in women, when menstruation is due to begin.

A purplish color is an indication that the symptoms of an aggravated heart and circulatory system were ignored and that the condition is growing more serious. It is often accompanied by chronically cold hands and feet, an indication of poor circulation.

A yellowish cast to the skin anywhere around the eyes indicates that the liver and gallbladder are overworked, usually from the excessive intake of cheese and other dairy products, although this condition is often seen in people who consume large amounts of carrot juice as well.

A grayish color around or under the eyes indicates malfunction of the lungs and kidneys, caused mainly by excessive consumption of heavy, fatty, dense animal foods as well as salt. Along with weakening lung and kidney function, the endocrine and lymph systems are growing sluggish. Not only caused by imbalances in the diet, this condition commonly arises from poor air conditions like those on airplanes and in high-rise buildings without proper ventilation systems.

Pimples anywhere around the eyes are the body's attempt to eliminate excess fat and protein. If the pimples are yellow, the excesses are more animal in origin, while red pimples arise from simple sugars. These pimples indicate that the kidneys, spleen, and lymphatic system are temporarily overworked from excessive eating of any kind.

The area of skin above the eyes and under the eyebrows is an indication of overall vitality. As we age, we worry obsessively about this skin sagging and growing puffy and loose. Erratic eating patterns and internal imbalance will cause this skin to deteriorate. The longer we remain imbalanced and overwork the body's various organ systems, the more quickly this skin will puff and sag. Altering our eating patterns in ways that nourish and serve us in our chosen lifestyle can keep this delicate skin strong and supple and even restore it to its former perfection.

Swelling or puffiness anywhere around the eyes indicates the pooling of liquid. The body, particularly the liver and kidneys, is unable to process toxins efficiently and so the excess accumulates.

Puffiness under the eyes seems to be the plague of modern people, right up there with dark circles. We have tried everything to reduce these puffy bags, even applying Preparation H (an unhealthy—and not recommended—use of this over-the-counter pharmaceutical) to this skin to shrink them, everything, that is, except altering the cause.

It used to be that puffiness didn't begin to occur until late adulthood, but it has become a problem for increasingly younger people. Bags under the eyes are caused by either pooled liquid or pooled mucus. Eye bags caused by either condition indicate chronic disorders of the kidneys, bladder, and other excretory functions. When the eye bags are caused by excessive fluid intake, they are often accompanied by frequent urination, as well as not sleeping well, both indications that the kidneys are overactive and aggravated.

When the eye bags are caused by excessive accumulation of mucus, they indicate that kidney function has grown sluggish, due to fat and mucus accumulating in the kidney tissue. When this happens, the kidneys can no longer absorb and discharge fluids and toxins from the body.

Eye bags are accompanied by a decline in our vitality. As the kidneys continue to overwork and weaken, we also weaken and grow chronically tired. Caused by the excessive consumption of fluids and animal fats, eye bags make us look as tired outside as we are inside. Simply balancing our intake of fluids and fats can restore our eyes to bright alertness and our kidneys to efficient function.

Double eye bags, which are commonly seen in the modern world, are caused by excessive intake of liquids and chemicals, like soft drinks and diet soft drinks. Double bags are a more serious version of the eye bags described above.

Wrinkled, crepelike skin under the eyes is an indication that the kidneys are growing dry and exhausted and are the result of excessive consumption of salt and animal proteins, as well as a lack of minerals (caused by a lack of them in the diet or the inability to absorb them into the bloodstream). A return to a balanced diet, rich in nutrients and variety will restore our eyes to their original glowing vitality.

The Nose

Ah, the noble nose. The nose reflects the health and function of the nervous system, circulatory system, and certain functions of the digestive system. It is said that the type of nose, size, shape, and other conditions reveal a great deal about character, as well as health.

It seems that all babies are born with cute button noses and as they grow, their diet, culture, and environment determine the final shape of each nose. A well-formed nose of average length, with slight roundness shows a balanced, stable character, with a strong ability to remain calm. A long, straight nose shows a more sensitive nature, while a shorter, flatter nose shows a tendency toward great determination. A larger nose indicates a capacity for great thinking.

The sides of the nose, reflecting the health of the liver, also show how we think. If the bones in the sides of the nose slope inward, making a graceful arc towards the tip, this shows a tendency toward clear, logical thinking. If the bones swell outward, this shows an ability to follow obscure thought patterns quite well.

Moving to the nostrils, they're more than how we breathe. Well-developed nostrils are said to reflect courage and determination. Less developed nostrils show a tendency towards timidity with a sensitive, creative nature.

Once the nose develops, each person is responsible for its condition. Life and diet choices influence its shape and size. Various changes in the normal shape of a nose indicate specific physical and mental conditions.

A high, sharp nose, often called an "eagle nose," is caused by the excessive consumption of poultry and eggs and shows that the arteries are hardening. This type of nose may also reflect a self-centered, restless nature.

If the tip of the nose tilts upward, this is caused by the excessive intake of fish and seafood, resulting in poor circulation, cold hands and feet, and a tendency toward shortsightedness in thinking.

A pointed nose, pointing strongly forward, is caused by the over-consumption of fruit and can result in diminished heart function with a tendency toward an excitable nature.

If the tip of the nose is swollen, like W. C. Fields, this is caused by many excesses in the diet, especially simple sugars, sweets, fats, and alcohol. This condition of the nose reveals an enlarged, weakened heart and a nervous, daring nature.

If the tip of the nose droops down, this reflects the excessive intake of raw foods and fruit and juices, resulting in weaknesses in the heart, kidneys, and bladder functions.

If the tip of the nose grows hard, this shows that the diet contains excessive amounts of saturated fats from animal foods, in particular, poultry, eggs, and cheese. This condition of the nose indicates that the arteries and muscles are hardening and fat is accumulating around the heart, liver, spleen, and pancreas.

A cleft in the tip of the nose is a sign of nutritional imbalance, specifically a deficiency in minerals. Caused by the excessive consumption of simple sugars and sweets that can deplete the blood of minerals, this condition can also be caused by chemical additives in the foods we choose. A cleft in the tip of the nose shows a tendency toward irregular heartbeat and is growing more common in these modern times, as we eat more and more foods not natural for us.

The color of the nose can be a clear gauge of our health and strength as well. If our health is balanced and vital, our nose is the same color as the rest of our face (sunburn notwithstanding). The quality of the skin will match the rest of the face, as will moisture or dryness. If the pores are enlarged or the skin is oily, for instance, that indicates a condition of imbalance.

If the tip of the nose is red, it shows that capillaries are expanding due to an excessive intake of liquid, alcohol, stimulants, and spices. This can indicate irregular blood pressure and a tendency toward hypertension. If the entire nose is red, the liver is also overworked and inflamed and is a more serious indicator of this imbalance.

If the nose should turn purple it is serious, because this is an indication that there is a tendency toward very low blood pressure and heart failure.

Expanded, broken capillaries in the skin of the nose indicate that the liver and heart are extremely overtaxed, with serious disorders of the heart and circulatory system on the horizon.

A pale, white nose demonstrates contraction of the heart and surrounding capillaries due to an excessive consumption of salt. It can also be caused by a diet devoid of vegetables and enough fluids. Along with this condition, you will usually find coldness in the extremities, cold, clammy skin, and a hesitant nature.

Pimples on the nose, as anywhere else on the body, are an attempt to eliminate excess. In the case of yellow or white pimples, the body is trying to discharge animal fats, specifically dairy foods. Reddish or dark pimples show the body attempting to discharge excessive amounts of simple sugar and sweets.

And should the nose accidentally be broken? An accident that damages the nose shows a weakness in the corresponding organ at the time of the break.

Nosebleeds are seen most often in children, as a way for them to discharge excesses, and for the most part they grow out of them. But as our diet degenerates, we see them more often in adults. In both men and women, they are an attempt by the body to discharge excess simple sugar and sweets. However, in the case of women, nosebleeds are most often seen in women whose menstrual periods are irregular and often disappear when the cycle normalizes. In men, a nosebleed indicates that they are growing internally weak from too many sweets, and a change in diet is needed. More strongly cooked foods with more minerals in the diet and far fewer sweets will return men to their normal strength.

The Cheeks

The cheeks, those lush bits of flesh that every Italian grandmother loves to pinch, those smooth orbs of skin that beg to be bussed, are meant to be irresistible. When the skin of the cheeks is clear and smooth, supple, and glowing with health, we know that the health of the respiratory and circulatory systems is doing just fine. Any irregularities in this skin of the face will show any number of imbalances that need attention.

If the skin on the cheeks appears very thin, with veins visible, this indicates poor balance in nutrition, particularly protein and fats. With this condition, you will usually also find weakness, shallow breathing, poor circulation, and an overly thin body. There are just not enough nutrients to keep the body functioning in strength.

Firm, tight flesh over the cheeks shows great physical strength, with very vital circulation and lung capacity. This appearance indicates deep vitality due to proper eating and exercise. Drooping cheek flesh, of course, would indicate weaker circulation and respiration, usually due to overeating and sedentary living.

Overall, the color of the cheeks should match the rest of the face without inflamed color, paleness, or other discolorations or marks.

Red or pink cheeks, except during exertion from exercise or in cold weather, is an indication that blood capillaries are abnormally expanded. Caused by the excessive intake of liquids, particularly soft drinks, chemicals, fruit juices, and sugary drinks, this condition shows that the heart and circulatory system are overworked and aggravated. With this condition, there may also be a tendency toward hypertension and an overly sensitive nature. Breathing may also be more shallow and faster than is normal, because the heart beat is quite rapid.

Milky white cheeks or cheek color that is more pale than the rest of the face is caused by the excessive intake of dairy foods, especially milk, soft cheeses, cream, and yogurt. Overeating of white flour products may also cause this discoloration, as can lack of aerobic exercise. In both cases, this condition shows the accumulation of fat around the lungs and large intestines and is often accompanied by sluggish, lethargic energy and can indicate anemia.

Pimples on the cheeks show the body's attempt to eliminate excess fat and protein accumulating around the intestines and lungs. Caused by animal foods, dairy foods, and saturated fats and oils, this condition can be chronic, changeable, and long lasting if our diet remains unchanged.

If the pimples are whiter in color, they are caused more by milk and simple sugar. If they have a yellowish cast, they are caused by eggs and cheese. Reddish pimples are caused by sugar and artificial chemicals and some drugs, including antibiotics, which can actually worsen the condition of acne. Pimples appearing in the center of the cheeks, with an inflamed and fatty appearance to them, are caused by fat hardening in various organs, possibly tending towards the production of cysts.

If a darker shade appears to be brushed across the cheekbone, this shows sluggish function of the kidneys and excretory system and is caused by the excessive consumption of simple sugar, in particular honey. However, this conditon can also be caused by too much salt in the diet. Both extremes overtax the excretory function.

If the cheeks take on an overall darker cast, it indicates a more serious weakening of the respiratory function and reduced lung capacity. Caused by chemicals and medications, this condition shows that there is blood stagnation in the lungs.

If the cheeks have a grayish cast, the liver needs attention. Excessive amounts of salt, animal protein, eggs, shellfish, and alcohol have caused the liver to move into overdrive. Often accompanied by a short temper, this condition shows that the liver and gallbladder are hardening from overwork.

Freckles on the cheeks simply show the elimination of sugar and sweets from the respiratory and digestive systems. Always harmless, freckles are the easiest way for the body to discharge any sugar it doesn't want.

Tiny hair on the cheeks, like fine silvery baby hair or down, indicates the excessive consumption of dairy products and shows that fat is accumulating around the reproductive organs. You may also see diminished lung capacity with this condition, as fat accumulates in the lungs.

A rosy, red color on the apples of the cheeks can be an indication of hypoglycemia, with blood sugar levels all over the charts. This condition can be caused by excessive intake of extreme foods, from protein to simple sugar. Most often, food is needed on a frequent basis to keep the condition stable. If the diet is adjusted to include whole grains, beans, and vegetables, minimizing simple sugars, utilizing complex carbohydrates, the blood chemistry will be stabilized over a relatively short period of time . . . and the cheeks restored to a normal color.

The Ears

The ears, those delicate shells that conduct the music of life into our lives, that love to be nibbled and kissed, reflect our entire physical and emotional condition but most especially the kidneys and their function.

The size and shape of our ears are determined while we are in the womb and are, therefore, constitutional and not likely to change in our lifetime. They do, however, reflect our inherent tendencies, strengths, and weaknesses and can help us to understand our health.

A balanced constitution shows itself as larger ears that begin at eye level and extend down to the mouth level and have a large lobe that is detached from the head. It is said that the larger the lobes, the longer your life and the stronger your vitality. Interestingly, if you look at our older generation, whose diet was more natural with less additives and processing, though not vegetarian, you will find many people with larger lobes, while most modern people have smaller lobes, since our diet is less natural and more imbalanced.

A bit of legend about the earlobe: It is said that in traditional societies, girls didn't pierce their ears until the age of nine (at the earliest), as it was believed that piercing the lobes stimulated the female side of our nature. It was thought that they would prematurely reach puberty and would sexually mature too early. Many cultures pierced girls' ears to indicate that they were ready for marriage and family.

Smaller ears show that the mother had an imbalanced diet during pregnancy, especially lacking in minerals, either due to simple sugar, which take minerals from the blood, or by not including mineral-rich foods in the diet. Eggs and meat can also cause this condition. These types of ears can indicate a more delicate character that works harder to maintain vitality. These people tend to be more conceptual in their thought patterns, and, while they have good vitality, it is only in short bursts.

Pointed ears are formed when the mother ate a large amount of animal protein not balanced by vegetables. These ears can reflect a more narrow-minded and stubborn nature and though they appear physically strong, these are people that tire easily as their internal organs are a bit weak from overwork since the womb. Ears that are positioned high on the head are also an indication that the mother consumed excessive amounts of animal food during pregnancy.

Thickly textured ears are the result of the mother having a proper, balanced diet and show a sound physical condition and emotional stability. Thin ears, on the other hand, are a sign of nutritional deficiencies and can indicate inherent weakness.

Ears that lay close to the head also indicate that the mother ate a properly balanced diet; ears that are slightly separated from the head indicate that the mother's diet was richer in raw vegetables and fruits; ears that stick out from the head can be caused by the mother consuming simple sugars, medications, and artificial chemicals.

The color of the ears has great import in showing our health. The ear is divided into three layers, inner, middle, and outer. The inner ear, the part of the ear that wraps around the actual opening into the ear, reflects the health and function of the digestive and respiratory systems. The middle ear, the area of the ear that is the largest scoop of the shell of the ear, reflects the health and function of the nervous system. The outer rim of the ear, the tougher flap that makes the perimeter, reflects the health and function of circulatory and excretory systems. The earlobe corresponds to the health of the kidneys and reproductive system.

Redness anywhere on the ears, unless it's cold outside or you are exerting yourself during exercise, indicates expanded blood capillaries and shows overwork and aggravation of the corresponding systems. Purple color anywhere on the ear, on the other hand, shows weak circulation and is usually accompanied by poor energy levels.

The Mouth

Oh, the mouth . . . kissable, seductive, smiling with luscious, moist, and inviting lips. This small area of the face gives us the ability to convey our messages, our sadness and our joy. With it, we can seduce or destroy. The mouth is needed to nourish and be nourished in so many ways, from physical food to affectionate cooing. Our mouths can also communicate volumes about us, without uttering a word. The mouth and lips reflect both the constitution and day-to-day condition of health and vitality. Specifically, the mouth and lips reflect the health and function of the digestive system and related organs. As the beginning of the digestive tract, the actual entrance for the food and drink we choose, the mouth very clearly shows the internal condition of the intestines.

As we have "modernized" our diets, the mouth has evolved. Just a few generations ago, the average, normal mouth was the same width as the nose, a reflection of an inherently strong and vital constitution. As our diets have changed to include more sugar, artificial chemicals, processed foods, and saturated fats, the average mouth has grown much wider, reflecting a more delicate constitution, with weaker organ function and a lower resistance to environmental changes and pollutants due to deficiencies of minerals in the diet from either chemicals and simple sugar or excessive protein, all of which leach minerals from the blood. The wider the mouth, the more delicate is the constitution of the person.

Different areas of the mouth and lips reflect specific organs, their functions, and health. The upper lip, for example, shows the health and function of the stomach, while the lower lip shows the health and function of the small and large intestines. Specifically, the middle portion of the lower lip shows the small intestine, while the peripheral area of the lower lip shows the condition of the large intestine.

The corners of the mouth reflect the health and function of the duodenum, specifically, with the right corner corresponding to the duodenum's reaction to the bile secretion of the liver and gallbladder and the left corner reflecting the pancreatic secretions.

Besides the constitutional and ancestral conditions of the mouth, whether a wide or narrow mouth, a bow mouth or thinner lips, the lips should be clear and uniform in color and size, with neither lip being substantially larger or smaller than its partner or than is normal for a particular culture.

There are several conditions of the body that will be reflected in specific conditions of the mouth and lips. Interestingly, these conditions will change slowly or quickly, depending on the diet and life choices we make to alter the disharmony in the body.

Pinkish, red lips show that the respiratory, circulatory, and digestive systems are working at their optimal best, with blood quality being strong and nourishing organ function to be its most efficient.

Overly vivid red lips indicate that the blood capillaries are expanded, suggesting high blood pressure and most likely, rapid breathing and racing circulation. Most often, however, you only see this color in the lips when the body is working to balance an infection or inflammation.

Whitish lips indicate strong constriction in the capillaries, which can be caused by anemia, sluggish circulation or blood stagnation. Whitish lips are most often caused by the excessive consumption of simple sugar and artificial chemicals, which weaken the blood, and dairy foods, which clog circulation, causing stagnation in the veins and arteries.

Dark lips are caused by sluggish circulation, specifically the blood plasma accumulating excessive amounts of fatty acids and salts. This constriction of the capillaries results in the dysfunction of the kidneys and urinary tract, and the liver and gallbladder begin to harden from overwork. Dark lips, with a reddish tinge to them, show excessive consumption of protein and saturated fats, as well as salt. Indicating weakening functions of the heart and circulatory system, this condition also shows weakening functions of the liver, spleen, gallbladder, pancreas, kidneys, and urinary tract. Basically, the body is showing signs of totally wearing down. Along with this coloring of the lips, you will most likely see an overall decline in vitality and physical strength and endurance.

Lips that are pale pink with a whitish tint show the excessive consumption of soft dairy foods, like ice cream and milk, sugar, and soft fats, like butter. Indicating a weakening of lymphatic function, this condition is often accompanied by allergies, tendencies toward skin eruptions, asthma, and hormonal imbalances.

A yellowish tint to the lips is the result of the excessive consumption of poultry, eggs, and hard cheeses. These kinds of dense, saturated fats cause the liver and gallbladder to harden and weaken in their ability to aid the body in the discharge of toxins.

The State of the Mouth

Clichés are always based on the truth. When we think of someone as closemouthed, the impression is strength of character, someone who can keep your secrets, not a gossip. On the other hand, loose lips sink ships. These two conditions of the mouth reflect our strengths and weaknesses.

Lips that naturally come together when at rest, gently closing the mouth, show that the nervous, circulatory, and respiratory systems are working soundly and efficiently.

A tightly closed mouth, with lips clenched, suggests that the liver, gallbladder, and kidneys are hardening from overwork due to the excessive consumption of meat, poultry, eggs, and salts.

Loose lips, on the other hand, or a mouth that, when relaxed, hangs open with lips parted, shows that the stomach, lungs, liver, gallbladder, and kidneys are growing swollen and weak, unable to contract and work efficiently due to the excessive consumption of raw foods, simple sugars, sweets, fruit juices, artificial sweeteners, chemicals, and even medications. Loose lips can also be an indication that, in general, a person is excessively consuming both food and drink.

Swollen lips, those "bee-stung" lips that enchant us so, actually show digestive disorders. A swollen, expanded top lip indicates chronic stomach trouble, usually the result of excessive amounts of poor quality food in the daily diet. The stomach is losing its ability to function efficiently. A swollen lower lip indicates intestinal difficulties, including chronic indigestion, constipation or diarrhea, and bloating. Just about seven out of ten people have swollen lower lips, showing that minor digestive disorders of the intestines are more common than those of the stomach. (When injections into the lips to make them appear full came into vogue, I was puzzled as to why a woman would want to look like she had digestive trouble when she didn't.)

If the mouth accumulates a crusty discharge at the corners, this shows the excessive intake of oily, greasy foods, which can affect the ability of the small intestine to function well. If the mouth is yellowish in color, the liver and gallbladder are excreting abnormal amounts of bile, due to the excessive consumption of saturated fats from meat, eggs, poultry, hard cheese, and fatty seafood.

A clearly defined mouth is the reward for not overeating or overdrinking. A clear, smooth, defining line around the mouth shows that digestion is sound, neither overworked nor undernourished. If the mouth is not clearly defined, it shows that digestion is overworked and that too much food is being consumed, even if the choices are healthy. This condition indicates that digestion is weak and tired from overwork, and the person has been indulging a bit too much.

Vertical lines that appear on the lips are an indication that hormonal function is receding and that sexual functions are declining. These lines usually occur later in life and many times in older people who are alone and not in a relationship. In younger people, these lines will usually appear if there is dehydration present from excessive consumption of salts and dry foods. These lines also occur in women who have had hysterectomies, particularly if the surgery was at a young age.

If the center of the lips, the delicate little dip in the center of the top lip is clearly shaped, this shows that the mineral balance in the bloodstream is in harmony. Indicating a balanced diet, this condition reflects strong, efficient functioning of the heart, small intestine, and reproductive system (including virility and desire). An ill-defined center dip in the upper lip, on the other hand, indicates that the heart, small intestine, and sexual strength are weaker, as the stomach and pancreas are overworking to process excessive amounts of sugars and fatty foods in the diet.

The Upper Lip

The upper lip, the skin just above the mouth, indicates the condition of our reproductive organs, as does the chin. Just like the face, this skin shows healthy sexual function when clear and smooth, matching the color of the rest of the face. Any abnormalities in this skin show a dysfunction in our reproductive system.

Reddish color indicates that the capillaries are expanded, due to the excessive intake of simple sugars, chemicals, and heat-producing spices, like cinnamon, curry, and cayenne. This condition is often seen in women with PMS, hot flashes, or painful menstruation. In men, this condition indicates that the prostate is aggravated and inflamed.

Pimples on the upper lip indicate that the body is eliminating accumulated fat and protein from soft dairy products, meat, and eggs.

If the upper lip takes on a grayish cast, particularly near the corners of the mouth, it indicates stagnant blood circulation due to the accumulation of fat around the ovaries in women and around the prostate in men. This discoloration is often seen in women whose menstrual cycles are irregular.

Hair on the upper lip has two very different meanings in men and women. In women, we don't want to see a moustache, even tiny fine hair. This indicates an excessive intake of protein, which causes fat to harden and accumulate around the ovaries and uterus. The hair is the body's attempt to discharge the excess protein and preserve the hormonal balance in the reproductive system. This condition can also be caused by overeating in general.

In men, strong facial hair indicates balanced production of testosterone and sexual virility. Understand, however, that in some cultures, strong facial and body hair is not the norm. For instance, most Asian men, Native Americans, many African American men, and some other cultures do not naturally have a lot of facial or body hair, so that differentiation must be made. In these cultures, the health of their testosterone production is seen in the uniformity of the hair growth. If the hair growth is patchy or irregular, it shows hormonal imbalance.

The Teeth

I have a Japanese friend who is perpetually perplexed by what he perceives as the American obsession with perfect teeth. He's right. We adore perfect teeth, a beautiful smile. Think Tom Cruise, Denzel Washington, and Julia Roberts. We wear braces, apply veneers, get caps, and bleach our teeth, spending billions of dollars on perfecting our smile. What is it about mega-watt smiles of white teeth that drive us to such lengths? The size, shape, color, and quality of our teeth show what we are made of, literally.

As children, we have twenty teeth and as adults, we have thirty-two. The shape and condition of our teeth indicates the quality of food consumed as we were growing and developing as children. While childhood dental care plays a role, food is the main source of health or disease of our teeth. The size, shape, color, pattern, and even number of teeth can vary depending on our childhood diets.

Adults generally have eight incisor teeth, four canines, eight premolars, and twelve molars. A full set of molars, however, doesn't grow unless the diet is well balanced. Often, an imbalance in the diet causes the third molars, the wisdom teeth, to develop abnormally, causing pain, and in some cases, they will not develop at all. The various teeth correspond to various organs and their function and can help us in diagnosing our health. The incisors reflect the health and function of the respiratory, circulatory, and glandular systems; the canines show the health of the liver, gallbladder, spleen, pancreas, and stomach; the premolars show the health of the upper digestive tract and the excretory system; the molars show the health of the small and large intestines and the reproductive system. This becomes important information when we consider dental work and decay. Decay in teeth indicates imbalances in the corresponding organs and their functions.

The pattern of growth of our teeth is a result of dietary choices made during the growing years and reflect a great deal about a person's tendencies, both physically and emotionally.

When the front teeth push outward, this indicates an excessive intake of raw vegetables, fruit, and juices, while the teeth were developing. Teeth that grow inward are an indication that the diet contained more animal foods, salt, and overcooked foods. Teeth that grow in different directions, some in, some out, overall more crooked, shows that the eating patterns were chaotic, with many extreme foods, bouncing back and forth between meat, eggs, poultry, cheese, and simple sugars, ice cream, soft drinks, chemicals, and alcohol. Think of how many modern people need braces to straighten crooked teeth. Then reflect on how much of the modern diet is centered on animal foods, processed foods, and junk foods. Legend has it that people with irregular teeth are prone to be quite fickle and changeable.

Teeth that are naturally straighter show that the diet is generally balanced nutritionally. We rarely see that occur naturally today. Most often, the teeth must be corrected.

Spaces between the teeth are the result of the jaws and gums expanding due to the excessive intake of simple sugars and artificial chemicals. If the spaces occur overall in the mouth, the condition is more delicate, with a tendency toward weakness. If the spaces occur between the two front teeth, it shows inherent weakness in respiratory and circulatory function. Italian folklore also says that space between the front teeth means that this person will grow quite wealthy in their lifetime, while in Asia, space between the front teeth indicates that the person will leave home at an early age.

The size of the teeth shows what foods were predominant in the diet as the teeth developed, with larger teeth being the result of larger proportions of protein, fat, and sweets, while smaller teeth show that the diet was richer in carbohydrates, minerals, and salt.

Many people are frustrated by abnormal surfaces on their teeth. Vertical ridges on the teeth are due to the excessive intake of salts and carbohydrates, with a deficiency of fat in the diet. Tiny pinholes in the teeth indicate a deficiency of both protein and vegetables, with an excessive amount of salt, and other minerals in our diet. If the front teeth have serrated edges on their bottoms, this is caused by an excessive intake of salt and not enough fat and protein in the diet.

Healthy, normal teeth will have a light ivory color, showing balanced organ function due to proper diet. Other colors will appear on the teeth as a result of poor eating habits, drinking, chemicals, and smoking.

A light yellow color is the result of poor dental hygiene, with the teeth staining because they aren't properly cleansed. A deeper yellow or dark brown color on the teeth is caused by smoking, tea, or coffee, whose acids can penetrate the enamel of our teeth and deeply stain them.

Gray color on the teeth is caused by a lack of dark, leafy green vegetables in the diet. This coloring on the teeth shows sluggish function in the liver, gallbladder, spleen, and pancreas, due to excessive intake of eggs, shellfish, and cheese. Gray color can also be caused by antibiotics taken during the developmental years of life, often appearing as gray stripes on the teeth.

A purplish color on the teeth is caused by an extremely excessive intake of simple sugar, specifically, fruit, juices, and chemical sweeteners. A purple color on the teeth can indicate that the respiratory function is weakening. Such an excessive amount of sugar in the diet will cause the lungs to expand but lose their ability to contract to expel air.

Teeth that chip or break easily is a condition caused by an excessive intake of salt, after years of excessive consumption of simple sugar and milk. The combination of extremes in the diet causes the teeth to become quite brittle.

If the teeth don't grow normally, especially during childhood years, it is the result of an imbalance in nutrition, but specifically, it is the result of the excessive intake of milk, even mother's milk. If taken for more time than is reasonable, milk will weaken the teeth's ability to grow. When an infant begins to grow teeth, it is the natural time to begin to wean from breast-feeding to solid food.

The cause of tooth decay is the excessive consumption of simple sugar and simple carbohydrates. Tooth decay occurs symmetrically, affecting the teeth in a specific pattern. If the upper left molar has decay, the upper right molar or lower left molar will also show decay. The thirty-two teeth correspond to the thirty-two vertebrae in the spine, which is how the connection between the teeth and the organ systems and glands of the body was made. When decay occurs then, it is usually accompanied by a weakening of the corresponding organ function.

Think about how tired you get after a dental visit. Because the teeth correspond directly to organ function, when the teeth are traumatized by the work being done, the corresponding organ will also feel the effects of the trauma. (And you thought it was just the anxiety of the visit to the dentist.)

Gums

Like the teeth and the mouth, the gums are reflective of specific conditions of our health. Normal gums are pink and firm, holding the teeth and setting off their respective colors to create a healthy, glowing smile.

If the gums are swollen and painful, this indicates that we are over-indulging in fats, simple sugars, fruit and juices, chemical sweeteners, and soft drinks.

Receding gums is an extreme condition caused by extremes in the diet. When the diet includes large quantities of meat, eggs, cheese, and poultry, as well as sugar, soft drinks, chemicals, chocolate, and honey, the gums will pull away from the teeth. This condition also naturally occurs with age.

Abnormally red or purplish gums, without swelling, are caused by salt and chemicals. If there is swelling, this condition is caused more by simple sugar and chemicals, rather than salt.

Pale, whitish gums are generally signs of anemia, caused by nutritional deficiencies.

Pimples on the gums or in the mouth cavity are the result of the body trying to discharge accumulating protein, fat, and oil, from both animal and vegetable sources.

Bleeding gums are caused by broken capillaries, which have been weakened by the lack of salt and minerals in the bloodstream, as well as from a lack of fresh vegetables in the diet.

The Tongue

More than the seductive pink sliver that slips between the lips, the tongue shows a lot about the physical and emotional constitution. In fact, the tongue is the window to your metabolic function. It is the only internal organ you can see. The shape, color, and texture of your tongue indicate the level of your vitality and ability to produce blood, which in turn affects your ability to digest food, breathe, eliminate toxins, and resist illness.

The shape of the tongue is determined by the foods consumed by the mother during pregnancy. A wider tongue is caused by more vegetable-quality food in the mother's diet during pregnancy and results in a generally strong, vital constitution and emotional stability. A narrow tongue with a pointed tip is caused by the consumption of more animal protein during pregnancy. While the constitution is healthy, this type of person is prone to muscle tightness in life, as well as having a more stubborn nature.

A flatter, thinner tongue is the result of a properly balanced diet during pregnancy, resulting in a strong, calm nature, while a thicker, coarse tongue is caused when the mother's diet during pregnancy tends to have more animal protein than vegetables and is said to produce a strong will.

The tongue is reflective of the health and function of the entire digestive system, with specific areas of it showing the condition of various organs.

The tip of the tongue reflects the health and function of the descending colon of the large intestine, with the periphery of the tongue showing the condition of the large intestine as a whole.

The center of the tongue shows the health and function of the small intestine, with the back edge of the tongue showing the condition of the duodenum, liver, gallbladder, and pancreas. The area of the tongue just to the rear of the center shows the health of the stomach, with the root of the tongue (behind the back edge) showing the condition of the esophagus.

The underside of the tongue shows the health and function of the blood and lymph circulation of each corresponding organ reflected on the top of the tongue.

The color of a normal, healthy tongue, showing that the digestive system is strong and efficiently working, is a rich pink. Any changes in the color of the tongue, specifically or overall, indicate a dysfunction in the corresponding organ or digestion as a whole.

If the tongue takes on a dark red color in specific areas, it indicates that there is an ulcer forming in the corresponding organ. If the color is an overall dark red, then the digestive tract is inflamed and aggravated.

A white coating anywhere on the tongue shows that circulation is sluggish, usually from the accumulation of fat in the digestive tract. It can also indicate anemia.

A yellowish color or coating on the tongue shows that the liver and gallbladder are secreting excessive amounts of bile, due to the accumulation of animal fat in the body, caused by meat, poultry, and eggs, specifically.

White spots or patches on the tongue are caused by the excessive intake of dairy foods and animal fats. This condition is indicative of an exhausted digestive system.

A blue or purplish cast to the tongue is caused by chemicals, drugs, and medication and indicates that circulation is tired and sluggish.

If pimples appear on the tongue, it shows the digestive tract eliminating excessive accumulations of animal protein, fat, and sugar. Pimples can also be caused by too much acid-producing foods in the diet, like citrus juice, acidic vegetables, alcohol, and poor-quality vinegars.

The Chin

"Not by the hairs on my chinny-chin-chin . . ." Hopefully, that little pig was a boy and not a girl, just one of the places females don't want to find any little hairs, but boys, on the other hand, as they become teenagers do.

Not just the part of the face used for resting on the hand, the chin reflects the health and function of the reproductive organs and, like the rest of the face, will have smooth, clear skin if the condition of the organs is healthy. Any irregularity or discoloration of the skin on the chin is an indicator that there is dysfunction in the reproductive system.

In women, if the chin is red, this is an indication that the blood capillaries have expanded due to the excessive intake of sugar and heat-producing spices, like cinnamon, curry, and cayenne. Usually, this condition is accompanied by strong PMS symptoms or hot flashes. In men, a red cast to the chin indicates an irritated and inflamed prostate, from the same causes.

In men or women, if the chin is irregular, dimpled, or with creases and lines, this indicates an accumulation of fat around the uterus or the prostate. In women, if a horizontal line appears across the chin, there is a tendency toward the formation of fibroids or a history of past fibroids. In men, the same kind of line indicates an enlarging of the prostate.

Pimples on the chin indicate that the body is trying to eliminate accumulating fat around the uterus, ovaries, or prostate, caused by the excessive consumption of meat, eggs, poultry, dairy foods, and sugar.

Hair on the chin is similar to hair on the upper lip, very different in men and women. In women, as on the lip, healthy reproductive function and hormonal balance is shown when there is no hair on the chin. In men, cultural implications considered, strong and uniform hair on the chin indicates hormonal balance and reproductive health.

REBALANCING YOUR GLOWING FACE

Now that you know what you're looking at in the mirror, what do you do? The art of seeing the condition of your health is a method of diagnosis that is meant to give you the power to be proactive in the creation and maintenance of your healthy life. Once you know what you are seeing, and what caused what you are seeing, it becomes easy to figure out how to rebalance any disorder to restore your natural radiant glow.

Natural facial care begins with daily food choices. The appearance of the face is a reflection of overall health and well-being. You are not doomed to premature signs of age, wrinkles, spots, lines, and creases. You don't have to live with pimples, splotchy color, and inflamed breakouts. The face can be a reflection of glowing health. With understanding and appropriate life and diet choices, you can look your very best.

The complementary areas of the body, internal and external, front and back, upper and lower, periphery and center are all parts of one whole being. These mirror images of each other are the key to your understanding. Whenever you experience a change on the inside, it is reflected on the outside. Visible, external signs, therefore, are an easy, accurate way for you to discern your condition and take appropriate action to change it to create what you want.

As we have just seen, dietary imbalances are the primary causes for the face not looking its best. Distortions of facial features, irregularities in the skin, abnormal growth of facial hair, and unwanted bumps and lumps can all be avoided by eliminating, or at least minimizing, extremes in the diet. Natural, appropriate food choices that are balanced for your condition are the most valuable cosmetics you can use. A balanced, well-prepared diet makes it so much easier to maintain your health, resulting in a youthful, glowing, vital appearance, in both face and body. Extreme foods, those foods that create excessive or depleting kinds of energy in the body, will disrupt the smooth flow of our life force—the energy that enlivens each being. For example, consuming a diet that is rich in fat and protein, meat, eggs, poultry, dairy foods, and hydrogenated oils causes the body's energy to sink and grow dense and stagnant. These kinds of foods overwork the body, as it struggles to maintain balance, weighted down with all these dense calories. On the other hand, a diet rich in sugar, chocolate, chemical additives, pesticides, fruit and juices, sodas, stimulants, coffee, alcohol, and hot spices can weaken the body as it struggles to hold on to energy, as these foods deplete it of nutrients and vitality.

Too many dense foods, such as dairy products and meat, cause us to feel heavy, lethargic, and tired, while too many dispersing foods cause us to grow weak, since we can't hold on to nutrients or energy. Either way, we lack the strength, stamina, and natural grace needed to glow with health.

This does not mean that extreme foods have no place in our diet and that life becomes a grim regime of doing only what is good for you. I live far too sensuously for that to be the case. If that were true, I'd probably change jobs to something more predictable and take my chances. Where we have gotten off the track to health is that we have completely forgotten what moderation means. If everyone consumed only small amounts of animal foods and even sugar, there would be no need for this book, because everyone would be glowing with health. Good health is about balance, not deprivation.

Once you have gotten yourself out of balance, however, and your glow is a bit skewed, what can you do to fix it and restore internal harmony? Rebalancing the various organ systems is done simply by understanding the nature of the organs involved, the foods that enliven them, and eating accordingly to restore your body's internal sense of balance.

In the Asian healing arts, organs are paired, denser with more hollow, yin with yang, for balance. In this method of diagnosis and healing, the organs are said to complement each other, functioning as a complete energy unit.

BALANCING THE ORGANS
Liver and Gallbladder

There are many ways of knowing that our liver and gallbladder are out of balance. Of course, we can look in the mirror and observe the tiny frown lines between our brows or an overall yellowish cast to our skin or the whites of our eyes. We can look at our temples and see if we have tiny, broken veins or a yellow color. We can also tell from our emotional state of health. Are we chronically cranky? Do we anger easily? All of these emotional responses to life's challenging situations are indications that the liver and gallbladder are aggravated and overworked, hardening in response to their exhaustion.

Balancing the liver and gallbladder to restore our healthy glow is as easy as understanding the energy of food and applying it accordingly. Foods with a delicate, ascending, expansive energy can help to restore balance to an overworked, exhausted, tight liver and gallbladder.

FOODS FOR BALANCING THE LIVER AND GALLBLADDER

Barley

Granny Smith apples

Leafy greens, especially bitter greens

Pickled and fermented foods, such as miso, soy sauce, sauerkraut, natural sourdough bread

Sour plums, vinegar, tempeh

Heart and Small Intestines

The heart and small intestines are enlivened by both extreme contracted energy and expansive energy. This is important to us because it explains why the heart and small intestines are so dramatically affected by extremes in our diet. Foods with extreme energies are particularly detrimental to the smooth function of the circulatory system.

In a healthy, normally functioning body, the arteries and blood vessels are open and flexible, making for clear, smooth circulation. If our diet includes too much animal protein and fat, the vessels grow stiff and clogged with accumulated deposits of fat and cholesterol, restricting circulation, causing the heart to overwork and exhaust itself. Foods with extreme contractive energy suppress the heart's natural function, distributing blood outward to all parts and organs of the body. When this constricted condition of the heart arises, the tip of the nose grows hard, as if cartilage is forming there, and we will experience a hardening of the collagen in the skin, showing up as hard, dry skin and arthritis-like symptoms in the joints.

On the other end of the spectrum, other foods that can adversely affect the function of the heart are strongly expansive foods, like sugar, alcohol, and chemicals. These foods, with their dramatic expansive natures, cause the heart muscles to weaken and the vessel walls to thin. Contributing to high blood pressure, enlargement of the heart, and mitral valve prolapse, the effects of these foods can be seen as an expanded tip of the nose, a reddened nose, or an overall reddish or splotchy complexion, caused by the dilation of capillaries.

Medical studies have shown a direct link between the excessive consumption of alcohol, sugar, and chemicals to deteriorating muscle strength and malfunction of the heart.

Situated at the deep center of the body, the heart sits near the center line of energy, meaning that its balanced function of expansion and contraction depends on the clear, smooth flow of both expanded and contracted energy through the body.

The small intestine is compatible, energetically, with the heart. Also located near the body's center line of energy, this portion of the digestive tract is dependent on the same rhythmic pulse of energy in the body to function smoothly.

Our digestive system is best suited to digesting plant foods. Our intestines are long and convoluted, while carnivores' intestines are shorter, relative to their size, allowing them to discharge animal protein and fat quickly, with little effort. For us, our long intestines cause the body to hold on to the toxins in animal foods, allowing them plenty of opportunity to break down into poisonous bacteria and other compounds, like ammonia. The toxic by-products of animal foods accumulate in the intestines, depleting the stock of friendly bacteria that live there, while saturated fats clog the capillaries in the villi, diminishing their power to absorb nutrients.

Strongly expansive foods, sugar, alcohol, and chemicals, cause the villi to expand and dilate, again, weakening their ability to digest and absorb nutrients. When this condition occurs, with the villi weakened and diminished in their capacity to absorb, we eat larger and larger amounts of food to obtain the nutrients we need to function and feel satisfied. We eat more and are able to use less food, resulting in being overweight. One of the most common side conditions to being overweight is nutritional deficiency.

FOODS FOR BALANCING THE HEART AND SMALL INTESTINES

Cooling vegetables (see list on page 28)

Corn

Cucumbers

Leafy greens

Pickled and fermented foods, such as miso, soy sauce

Sea plants

Spleen, Pancreas, and Stomach

Considered in Chinese medicine to be the center of our being, the spleen, pancreas, and stomach are enlivened by energy that gathers and holds, rather than by energy that disperses itself. What these organs crave, as the very core of our stability, is balance.

When our spleen, pancreas, and stomach are properly enlivened and functioning at their best, we feel centered and secure. We experience less anxiety, feel more focused, calm, and confidant. We are able to step outside ourselves and feel compassion for others and their feelings. We are thoughtful and able to maintain our sense of direction in life.

If the spleen, pancreas, and stomach grow unstable, it's as though the rug has been pulled out from under us. We feel so unsure of ourselves that we become self-centered and paralyzed. Over time, we will develop a suspicious nature and lose our ability to achieve our goals.

As the spleen, pancreas, and stomach grow imbalanced, our face changes, with a horizontal ridge forming at the top of the bridge of the nose. If the imbalance continues, we will lose our animation, the light in our eyes, and expressive emotion. Even when speaking, we will talk in more of a monotone, with little or no expression in gesture, eyes, or face. We will also be prone to weight gain, growing lethargic, depleted of energy, unable to get it together.

Relocating the center is easy. A balanced, stable diet is the key to calm serenity. The spleen and pancreas are solid, compact in structure, enlivened by gathering energy. And even though the stomach is hollow and more expanded, it is compatible with the spleen and pancreas and is also enlivened by a more contracting energy.

FOODS FOR BALANCING THE SPLEEN, PANCREAS, AND STOMACH

Brown rice syrup, barley malts, amasake (all whole-grain sweeteners)

Sweet ground vegetables, such as onions, cabbage, winter squash

Millet

Pears, peaches, and sweet apples

Sweet root vegetables, such as carrots and parsnips

Sweet brown rice

Lungs and Large Intestines

Without air, we no longer exist and without digestion of food, we no longer exist. The lungs and large intestines are responsible for our strength. They are largely responsible for how we present ourselves, striding confidently forward or without the courage to walk into a room alone.

The lungs are dense organs, packed with blood vessels and alveoli (tiny air sacs). Their compact structure is balanced by the hollow structure of the large intestine, which is a long, open tube, wound and packed into a tight space. Both of these organs cover the left and right sides of the body and are enlivened by contracted, intense energy. The intestines govern the function of the lungs. Without strong intestinal function, the lungs grow weak. The core of our strength lies in the large intestines.

They govern our ability to act on our desires. We've all heard the clichés "gutsy" and "gutless." These expressions are based in truth. We either have deeply rooted strength or we don't, and it shows.

The large intestines are responsible for (among other things) the regulation of moisture in the body. If the intestines grow wet and congested, the lungs grow wet and congested, decreasing lung capacity. If the intestines grow tight, hard, and dry, so do the lungs, without enough moisture to function well. From this condition, symptoms of asthma can arise. So the job of managing moisture in the body is paramount to the smooth function of the lungs.

Alike energies repel each other, like trying to put two north ends of a magnet together. Since the lungs and large intestines are contracted, by nature, they are quite sensitive to the effects of constricting energy.

Extreme foods like meat, eggs, salty cheese, and poultry will overwork and exhaust the large intestines and depress their function. On the other hand, the intestines need contractive energy to maintain strength and vitality. The overconsumption of sugar, chemicals, chocolate, soft drinks, and acidic vegetables and fruits will cause the intestines to grow swollen and flaccid, depressing their ability to contract and expand equally, pulsing with life. Dairy foods, like milk and soft cheese, will cause the accumulation of sticky mucus in the large intestines, diminishing our ability to absorb oxygen and discharge waste products. When the lungs and large intestines grow weak or clogged, we look stale and pasty, with dull skin, lifeless hair, and brittle or fragile nails. To maintain the strength of the intestines, stability is the key.

Energetically speaking, the differences between plant and animal foods are quite vast. In these terms, protein is not just protein, and there's a difference between plant-based fats and dense animal fats. The nutrients in plants are quite stable and break down slowly and efficiently in the body, while animal-based nutrients are inefficient fuel, unstable and requiring tremendous amounts of our resources to process them.

The rates of colon cancer among people who consume a great deal of animal protein, with less plant fiber, are substantially higher than in people who rely more heavily on plant foods, with less animal protein and fat. As a species, we eat about one-fifth of the vegetable fiber we did a hundred years ago and as our animal food consumption rose and grain and vegetable consumption reduced, we saw an epidemic rise in degenerative disease. Coincidence? I think not.

FOODS FOR BALANCING THE LUNGS AND LARGE INTESTINES

Brown rice

Burdock

Kuzu

Lotus root

Root vegetables with tops, especially carrots, daikon, and parsnips

Sea plants

Kidneys and Bladder

The kidneys and bladder house and protect our deepest life force, nourishing and supporting our vitality. Considered in Chinese medicine to be the core of our being, the kidneys and bladder govern our survival instinct, our courage, and are considered to be the root of our will and the seat of our sexual vitality and function.

Of primary concern in this area of the body is the health and function of the adrenal glands (situated just above the kidneys). The adrenal glands govern the function of our instinct, how we respond to perceived threat, working hand in hand with the kidneys. Filtering toxins from the blood, the kidneys also balance the electrolyte level in our bloodstream, determining the level of responsiveness of our nervous system. Together, these organs determine how we perceive threat and how we respond— reacting or overreacting.

If the kidneys, bladder, and adrenals grow weak or depleted, we perceive everything around us as a threat and grow tentative and fearful in our approach to life, including relationships with romantic partners. When these organs are overworked and exhausted, we begin to display signs of nervous energy, maybe even tics or twitches. We grow self-protective, with our arms crossed over our chests to shield our perceived vulnerability to attack.

Our skin takes on a decidedly washed out, pale cast, with deep blue patches under the eyes. We may experience chronic back pain, puffiness under the eyes, swollen feet and ankles, and tendency toward weepiness.

To restore the health and function of the kidneys and bladder, we have to understand their energy. The kidneys have a solid, compact structure, which is balanced by the more hollow structure of the bladder. The kidneys are situated in both the right and left sides of the body and are therefore considered, in Chinese medicine, to have a floating energy, not dominated by downward or upward movement, but rather supported by a balance between the two.

Dietary extremes take a great toll on these hardworking organs. Dense animal fats and proteins will clog the network of nephrons (tiny capillaries and specialized cells), inhibiting the kidneys' ability to filter and cleanse the blood. In addition, uric acid and other toxins produced by animal fats will build up around the kidneys and can damage the delicate cells that comprise the kidneys. On the other end of the "fat spectrum," the excessive consumption of sugar and sweets will turn into fat and accumulate around the kidneys, again, inhibiting their ability to function.

Fluids, in general, can have a tremendous effect on the kidneys and bladder and their function. Excess consumption of liquids causes the kidneys to overwork and grow exhausted, eventually washing away nutrients as well as waste in the blood. Drinking lots of water to flush the system of toxins is only helpful when our diet consists of many toxic foods. When we eat properly and drink only as needed, flushing the system is unnecessary, since the body is naturally taking in and discharging waste as needed to function well.

Sensitive to salt, the kidneys and bladder work best when good-quality salts are used in moderation in our diets. Natural sea salts, with very little processing, are the best for the health of our kidneys. However, even with superior salts, if excessive amounts are consumed, the kidneys grow tight and dry, causing the body to retain fluid, with swelling and a puffy appearance plus an overall tightening of the muscles in the body, particularly the lower back.

Excessive activity can also put a strain on the kidneys and bladder. Standing for very long periods, working under extreme conditions, either intensely hot or cold, or excessive exercise all can put a strain on the health and function of these organs. Too much, too cold, or too little fluid in the case of activity can exhaust these organs that love balance.

FOODS FOR BALANCING THE KIDNEYS AND BLADDER

Adzuki Bean Tea (page 308)

Burdock

Kasha

Miso

Sea plants

Sea salt

Shiitake Tea (page 309)

Smaller beans that are lower in fat, such as azuki beans, lentils, black turtle beans, and chickpeas

Soy sauce

THE GLOWING CYCLES OF RADIANCE

As we have seen, the energy that nourishes the body is ever-changing and flowing, inward, outward, ascending or descending, ebbing and accelerating, all working in concert to enliven our bodies to function at their greatest potential, bringing out the best in all of us. Influenced by many factors, diet, lifestyle, and environment, these energies are also influenced by forces much greater than broccoli and need to be considered when thinking about our health and vitality.

Types of Energy

Upward energy, the energy of morning and spring, enlivens and vitalizes the liver and gallbladder. They respond so well to being lifted and opened, since their job can leave them heavy and contracted.

Expansive energy, the energy of noon and summer, enlivens and vitalizes the heart and small intestine. These organs rely heavily on activity to stimulate the circulation so vital to their work in the body.

Downward energy, the energy of late afternoon and Indian summer, enlivens and vitalizes the spleen, pancreas, and stomach, our center of strength. This gathering energy pulls our resources toward our center, helping us to remain calm and focused, while preserving our energy.

Condensed energy, the energy of evening and autumn, enlivens and vitalizes the lungs and large intestine. Without energy deep in the body, the intestines can't efficiently do their job, leaving the lungs short of resources.

Floating energy, the energy of the night and winter, enlivens and vitalizes the kidneys and bladder. These organs, the very core of our strength and potential, store our resources for distribution as we need them. This dormant energy helps them to hold and store our precious strength.

Seasonal Changes

Let's look at seasonal changes and times of the day. How these factors influence our appearance can be quite interesting.

Within seasonal changes, we can see how energy affects our appearance. Warmer weather in spring and summer causes us to take in more fluids, and the strong expansive energy of these seasons moves our body fluids to the periphery of the body, causing us to sweat. Excessive intake of fluid and sweets can leave us with oily skin and pimples that worsen in the heat of summer. We compound the trouble with excessive use of air conditioning, drying the skin, causing oil production to increase even more.

Choosing, for the most part, a diet that is naturally balanced within seasons and daily cycles creates the most solid foundation for preserving our radiant glow. A varied diet, based on a wide range of seasonal ingredients, as well as varied cooking methods, makes it easier to transition smoothly and naturally through life. A balanced diet strengthens us and our day-to-day condition, pooling our resources and creating a deep well of energy to draw on for our lifestyle. Minimizing imbalances (we can never prevent them) and eating well result in a fresh, vital appearance, reflecting our internal strengths. Honoring the changes in the energies of the seasons and the day will leave us looking our best from morning to night, from spring to winter.

Spring: Springtime represents the beginning of expansive energy in the world. A time of renewal, new vegetation appears, with pale, cool greens dominating the color of the landscape. Plants begin to sprout upward, opening to growth. We begin to venture outward as well, lifting winter weary faces toward the sun.

Summer: Showing itself as the peak of expansive energy, summer with its hot sunlight and warm temperatures encourages abundant growth in the plant kingdom, making for a very active environment, for plants and for us, as we spend more time out of doors, in the sun, actively moving. During the end part of summer, Indian summer, we begin to see changes in nature, as plants begin to gather their energies inward, preparing for the dormancy of autumn and winter. At harvest time, we begin to also gather our resources for the months ahead.

During the summer, with our higher activity levels and the warm weather, we tend to consume more expansive foods to balance the contracting energy of heat. Excessive consumption of these kinds of foods, sugar, fruit, juices, and alcohol, can cause broken capillaries in the skin, giving us a reddish color or red nose, while expansion in the intestines and stomach can cause us to have puffy lips.

Autumn: Autumn displays the most contracted, dense energy. Leaves drop from plants, as they pull their life forces into their roots for winter storage. We turn more inward as well, spending less time outside, returning to school, studies, and indoor gatherings.

Winter: With winter, we experience a kind of dormant, expectant energy, floating somewhere between passive and active, witness to the plant world's quiet, watchful peace; all the world is waiting for the winter solstice, the signal that we have turned the corner back toward the light of spring, as slowly increasing sunlight activates the energy of the coming season. With the arrival of spring, energy blossoms once again and the cycle continues.

Cold temperatures and condensing energy cause the skin to dry and contract in the autumn and winter, leaving it tight and flaky. With oil glands naturally more sluggish in cooler weather, as well as living in the drying atmosphere of indoor heating, we can find our skin and hair demanding moisture.

In both these instances, we can counterbalance the unnatural environments we have created with green plants in our homes. These houseplants have the ability to balance the atmosphere by enriching the oxygen content of our air. Opening the windows for short periods will also help to normalize our environment.

In colder weather, our consumption of stronger protein, oil, and salt can result in sluggish, dry, dull skin, as fats clog the pores, compromising its ability to discharge toxins and absorb moisture. These kinds of foods have a sinking, condensed character and prevent our energy from rising to nourish our upper organs, particularly the liver, creating a tendency toward deeper and longer-lasting lines between the brows.

Daily Energy Cycles

Time of day isn't all that different from the changing seasons, energetically speaking. In the morning, ascending energy is most dominant, as the sun rises and we rise and begin our day's activities. By noon, the energy of the day is at its peak, as we are, moving actively through the world. As afternoon wears on, energy begins to gather and sink. We begin to tire and pull our resources inward to fuel us for the rest of the day. With evening, energy becomes most condensed, with the setting sun and gathering darkness. Our energy is at its most heavy, preparing for rest. Think of how weary we are as we travel home in the evening after a day's activity. During the night, the world's energy rests, as we do, floating between dormancy and expectance of morning. As morning approaches, the world's energy begins to move and open. We rise and the cycle continues.

These cycles of energy affect the body in very specific ways, enlivening the organs most receptive to energy at certain times of the day and year. Our appearance is strongly affected by these cycles. Our face, skin, hair, and overall vitality depend on our ability to work in sync with these energies. Body fluids take on the tendency to float and disperse toward the head and the periphery of the body at night when we sleep. This results in our skin looking fresh and plump in the morning. We look rested and refreshed, wrinkles and lines seem to diminish if our internal organs and energy are balanced. If, however, our organs are overworked and exhausted from too much liquid, fat, and sugar in the diet, our skin will stretch during sleep, resulting in puffiness and eye pouches as our body fluids pool and collect.

On the other end of the spectrum, as the day wears on, we lose moisture from perspiration and activity. This causes the cells and organs to contract and dry. If our diet is imbalanced, with excessive consumption of saturated fats and salt, dry skin can feel especially tight later in the day, leaving us looking drawn and worn.

During the late afternoon, it's natural for our energy to flag a bit, as our blood sugar levels take a dip. This is the time when energy begins to sink and condense, so it becomes difficult for us to maintain a high energy level. As we struggle to continue to expend great amounts of energy, we find ourselves growing exceedingly weary and begin to crave sweet taste to help us gather our resources for strength. All of this is natural. Where we cross the line and begin to move toward hypoglycemia is on those occasions where we feed those natural needs with sugar, artificial chemicals, or coffee. Treating this natural condition of settling energy with excessive amounts of sugar and stimulants, we are unable to stabilize our blood chemistry, tending to overeat and gain weight. In addition, a hypoglycemic condition can result in eczema and skin allergies, as well as triggering the release of androgens that activate oil-producing glands, which can result in oily skin and pimples.

As night folds around us, the natural tendency of energy is to move downward and inward. We journey home, gather together, and begin to ready the body for rest. Our skin, organs, and cells draw vitalizing energy from the environment as we rest, rejuvenating and recharging us. Working against these natural cycles, like choosing foods that have a strong expansive energy, wreck havoc on our appearance. Coffee and other stimulants accelerate strong upward energy in the body, stimulating the upper organs and brain, making it difficult to rest as we should, which leaves us looking less than our best. Lack of sleep will also divert blood circulation away from the face and skin, leaving us looking as drained as we feel, pale and hollow, with dark circles under our eyes, as the kidneys grow exhausted from lack of rest.

Honoring the changes in the energies of the seasons and the day will have us looking our best from morning to night, spring to autumn.

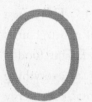

Your Glowing Skin

Our skin, if soft, smooth, and dewy, is the pride and joy of our bodies, or if not, it is the plague of our beauty regime. Glowing, healthy skin doesn't just happen but is the result of healthy, balanced life and diet choices. The skin, the largest breathing organ, is so easy to maintain and yet we struggle endlessly—and usually futilely—to create the appearance of health. Simple, balanced eating and living is what creates the supple, flawless skin we all desire.

In keeping with the philosophy of balance between expansion and contraction, the skin, the most peripheral organ of the body, reflects the condition of its complementary partner, the internal environment and the condition and function of our various organ systems. Remembering that the main function of the skin is to regulate the internal function of the body with the external environment, it will also mirror any environmental changes we experience. For instance, if we spend time in the sun, the skin darkens to protect our delicate internal organ systems. If we grow cold, the skin dries, so that the body can release moisture and warm itself internally.

When we see a flawless, glowing complexion, we are perceiving skin on more than just the physical level. Obviously, we are enamored of the clear, smooth appearance of this deliciously supple skin, but we are also feeling a quality of freshness, radiance, and vitality that transcends the physical characteristics of skin. We are seeing, on the skin, a reflection of health and aliveness. It is the combination of the physical and energetic qualities of someone's health that makes the strongest impact on us.

Glowing skin is more than skin deep, however. The health of our skin is the result of smooth, efficient organ function, which is the result of the life force that runs through us. What is life force? It's nothing that you can touch or smell, but it's as real as anything you can hold in your hand. Life force is the energy from the sun, earth, water, and sky that enlivens us, that charges our bodies with the vitality of nature.

In order to maintain naturally glowing skin throughout life, we need to understand the factors that encourage—and inhibit—the flow of energy through the body. We must begin to determine how the choices we make every day affect the life that moves through us. The easiest way to see how energy affects us, and to see results of our efforts, comes from something over which we have control, our food. Our food is what creates the blood and body fluids that nourish and create everything that makes us . . . us. If our food choices are fresh and vital, the energy that they conduct to our cells via our blood will be reflected in a fresh, vital, glowing appearance, beginning with flawless, lush skin. Our skin is the most peripheral area of the body and is a reflection of our total health. What we choose to eat and drink, as well as our choice of lifestyle, exercise and activities, are the most important factors that combine to conduct energy through our bodies smoothly and actively, creating overall good health and glowing skin.

Complex carbohydrates are great sources of fiber, which promotes smooth function of the intestines and digestive tract, which when functioning smoothly, ensure that waste products are eliminated from the body regularly. If the importance of that escapes you, just watch a laxative commercial and pay attention to the before and after scenes. Before taking the laxative, the poor constipated subject is dejected and lethargic, but after, is brimming with vitality, running about the yard with his dog. We can achieve this same vitality without harsh chemicals by simply consuming fiber in our diets. Your skin will glow with health, since there won't be any stagnating waste accumulating in various places of the body, making skin look lifeless and dull.

Whole, natural foods are also powerhouses of nutrition. Packed with vitamins, minerals, trace elements, protein, carbohydrates, and even some fat, these types of foods literally fill our reservoirs with energy, keeping us well-stocked with fuel to burn. With a strong foundation, we can go through life gracefully, rarely look washed out and tired, with dull, lifeless skin. Of course, we'll tire after a day's activities, but a night's sleep will find us refreshed, with soft supple skin to face the day.

So what doesn't work for us? What foods rob us of the supple, lush, touchable skin we are meant to have? To answer that, we need to look at our modern lifestyle, as well as eating habits—there's more than our food at the center of it, but it begins with our diet.

THE SKINNY ON SATURATED FAT AND CHOLESTEROL

In most of the industrialized world, fat accounts for 40 to 45 percent of our daily diets. Yikes! However, we need fat in moderation for normal body function. Saturated fats (and cholesterol), like those found in hamburgers, pizza, fried foods, dairy products, meat, eggs, and the ever-popular snack foods, accumulate around various organs, clog blood vessels, and inhibit body functions. The result is that the flow of vitalizing energy is inhibited and blocked, leaving the body hard and inflexible and our skin looking tired and dull as the pores grow blocked with accumulated fats, making it difficult to take in moisture and release toxins as needed. At this point, the skin accumulates layers of dry, dead cells, which make it look dull, tired, and in need of a good exfoliation. Excessive consumption of these fats is the culprit for scaly shins, heels, and elbows, making these conditions the greatest boon for the loofah industry, as we struggle to recover our skin's life, as well as our body's life.

It's easy to see how excessive consumption of saturated fat and cholesterol contributes to our internal demise, but now take a look in the mirror. Little lines between the brows? Dark circles under the eyes? Tight, dry skin—or an oily "T-zone"? Look a bit harder and older than you should at your age? All these conditions of the skin and face that plague us are the result of accumulated, hardened fat and cholesterol throughout the body. Choosing these kinds of foods prematurely ages and wrinkles the skin as they cause our various organ systems to overwork and exhaust themselves.

VISIONS OF SUGARPLUMS DANCED IN THEIR HEADS

While it sounds lovely in a fairy tale, simple sugars create anything but a happy ending for our skin and overall health. Simple sugars, from those sparkling little crystals to fruit and juices, are simple carbohydrates, and the difficulty lies in the amount of simple carbohydrates that we consume versus the amount of complex carbohydrates.

Sugar is found, of course, in the obvious places, candies, chocolate bars, soft drinks, and other snack foods. I can hear many of you saying, "But I don't eat that stuff." Just read a few labels. Sugar is an ingredient in so many other products, from breads and pasta to cereals to salad dressings and sauces and other processed foods, that we are consuming tremendous amounts of simple, refined sugar without actually eating junk food. And if you think shopping in a natural-food store is your salvation, think again. In most cases, you'll still need to read labels as diligently as you do in any supermarket. From maple syrup, high fructose corn syrup, fructose, sucrose, molasses, and honey to organic cane juice, which is just a fancy name designed to disguise sugar, many natural products contain as much simple sugar as any snack you can pick up in a convenience store.

Sugars are rapidly absorbed into the bloodstream, causing the glucose level to rise very quickly. When this happens, the pancreas (the organ that regulates blood sugar) secretes insulin that moves excess sugar from the blood to the cells. With this, blood sugar drops, resulting in rapid fluctuations in metabolism, what we know as sugar "highs" and "lows," as the levels of glucose in the blood rise and fall erratically. We experience a burst of energy as the levels of glucose rise, followed by the inevitable crash, as the glucose levels drop, leaving us feeling depleted and tired.

If we continue this pattern over time, the body grows exhausted from the extreme levels of energy, as well as the sugar robbing our bones, teeth, and skin of essential minerals, leaving us looking as tired and burned out as we feel. It gets even worse with sugar. Causing the expansion of capillaries of blood vessels near the surface of the skin, simple sugar is the major cause of skin discoloration—from freckling to red blotches to large brown "age spots." This discharge of excess energy depletes the body on several levels, robbing the body of calcium and other essential minerals, contributing to the loosening of tissue and muscle, leaving us looking weak and puffy, not to mention overweight and lethargic.

THE SALT OF THE EARTH

A necessary ingredient to life, salt has two very different sides to its nature. Literally vital to our existence, natural salt (sodium chloride) is rich in trace minerals that are necessary to the health of our blood. On the other hand, there's processed, refined table salt, the kind found in snack foods like potato chips, popcorn, salted nuts, and processed foods and meats. Table salt, far removed from its natural state in the sea, has been stripped of nutrients, re-enriched with iodine, and laced through with additives. In this state, even small amounts of salt will have a most dramatic effect on our blood chemistry and organ health.

Salt has a job in cooking—to make food taste like itself; we miss it when it's not there. Applied to food, salt causes contraction, sealing in the flavor of each ingredient, while forcing liquid from the food, intensifying the taste. It works similarly in the body. Consumption of natural salt, in appropriate quantities in cooking, aids the body in staying strong, with healthy blood, as our muscles and body tissue contract slightly. Used well, natural salt can also help our skin hold its precious moisture and retain its elasticity and firmness.

Excessive use of any salt, even sea salt, will have a dramatic effect on how we feel and look. Inappropriate use of salt or poor quality salt will cause tissue in the body to tighten and constrict, inhibiting the flow of blood to our various organs. Energy flow is blocked and we begin to feel tightening throughout the body. Our muscles begin to contract, growing stiff and hard. Our skin dries and tightens and will show signs of wrinkling long before it is natural to see those lines of experience.

Over time, should excessive use of salt continue, we will also see signs of degeneration in our bones, as the salt dries the body, inhibiting the absorption of vitamins essential to bone health and strength. We will lose our ability to stand tall and straight, as our bones grow brittle and weak.

Does this mean that to be beautiful, we're doomed to a grim regime of foods with no sparkle? No. Moderate use of salt, in cooking, not only adds to the pleasure of eating food, but starts the process of digestion, causing the food to soften as we apply the heat of cooking. Natural, unrefined sea salt, naturally aged soy sauce, and miso are the best choices for use of salt. However there should be no additional salt or soy sauce added to cooked food at the table. Raw salt, added to food, will only succeed in making our muscles tight and hard, our skin dry, and our joints inflexible. However, used delicately in cooking, salt makes eating a pleasure, our blood healthy, our muscles strong, and our skin firm and elastic. A sprinkle a day . . .

WATER, WATER EVERYWHERE . . .

In our culture, it's not uncommon for people to consume tremendous amounts of liquid every day, several cups of coffee or tea, soft drinks so large they could double as swimming pools, fruit juices, alcohol, eight glasses of water—or more. This kind of liquid consumption far exceeds the body's natural need for moisture.

However, we crave more and more liquid as a result of less and less natural eating. As we consume more salt and animal protein, hard fats and simple sugar, we need the moisture to balance the body. As the salt tightens the muscles and tissue, we take the liquid to soften and relax the body. As the protein produces internal heat as the body works to digest, we crave liquid to put the fire out and cool us down. Simple sugar is so strong in the body that we crave moisture to dilute its effect. While it sounds like we are simply making balance—and in truth, we are—it's the kind of balance that has us bouncing, yo-yo–like, from one extreme to the other, exhausting our reserves and leaving us looking tired and depleted. And there's more.

Excessive consumption of liquid expands and loosens the tissue of the body, weakening its ability to conduct our valuable life energy to all its parts. Increasing the amount of liquid in the circulatory system, excessive fluid in our diet overworks the heart, kidneys, bladder, and sweat glands, causing us to feel weak and tired, with loose skin and a "washed out" look, because, we are exactly that, washed out.

If excessive consumption of liquid continues over time, our body grows flaccid and our facial features lose definition. In fact, as excess liquid in our system causes the skin to puff, wrinkles in the forehead and under the eyes will deepen and increase, with the icing on the cake being puffy bags under our tired eyes.

Of course, the body needs fluid to survive. Without sufficient liquid, our skin tightens and dries and our organs grow constricted. Drinking for comfort is the best rule of thumb, with attention paid to diet and lifestyle. If you live an active life, you will require more liquid than someone more sedentary. If you work on computers for long stretches of time, you will find yourself feeling more thirst. If you tend to eat salty or sweet foods in excess, you will need more fluid to balance your internal environment. Consumption of too many dry foods or baked foods will also leave you feeling parched more often.

Balance, of course, is the key. The body will have it, and your cravings are the proof. Most of us, even if eating a relatively healthy diet, spend a great deal of time in extreme states, either flooded with excess liquid, as described here, or dehydrated. Ironically, we can be drinking great amounts of liquid and still feel dry and parched. Tea, coffee, fruit juice, soft drinks, and alcohol, while wet, dehydrate the tissue of the body, either from their sweet taste or diuretic natures. Water, taken in to our comfort, is the best source of moisture for the body, with other liquids consumed for pleasure but not for thirst quenching.

On top of fluid intake, diet plays a significant role in the level of our thirst. Consumption of dry foods, animal protein and fat, sweets, salt, and baked foods will leave us perpetually parched. On the other hand, a diet of whole grains, soups, beans, and vegetables is rich in moisture that the body can absorb and store in a balanced state. Because of their moisture content and fiber, a diet based largely on plants keeps our bodies nicely hydrated and thirst is based more on lifestyle and activity. Drinking for thirst and pleasure, rather than habit or craving, will keep our skin supple and soft and our appearance alert and vital.

We've all seen the effects of too little protein on humans. Excessively thin, with a hollowed out, sunken-in look, people who lack protein in the diet usually end up with loss of muscle and overall weakness. However, for most of us, our problems with health and appearance come from too much protein, rather than too little.

In adults, the primary requirement of nutrition is to create fuel to carry us through our daily activities with the secondary job of forming and maintaining cells (the primary job of nutrients in children). That means that we require fuel that can be efficiently burned to keep our fires lit. In general terms, complex carbohydrates are the burning fuel, with protein used to repair, construct, and maintain tissue. So naturally, we can conclude that, as adults, most of us require more carbohydrate energy than protein energy to sail through our days. In our modern way of eating, however, protein has become the star of the show with carbohydrates being neglected, even denigrated.

We require protein for strength and for the maintenance of our muscles. Without it, we grow weak, with sunken cheeks and an overly thin body. Without sufficient protein, our body will begin to feed on its own muscle for maintenance and strength. But how much is enough—and when is it too much? I find it interesting that, with all we know of nutrition, we are still quite perplexed by protein and how much we require. We have no explanation, for instance, as to why everyone seems to require differing amounts to be comfortable and healthy. Why do some of us require protein at both lunch and dinner to maintain our energy level, while others will fall promptly asleep after a protein lunch, feeling lethargic and sluggish? I think that protein is quite personal and that we must look at our lifestyles, activity levels, and needs to decide how much protein we need to maintain our vitality.

While protein is quite important to our nutrition and maintaining our vitality, we must understand it. As with everything in nature, there is a front and back to the wonder food—protein. Compared to carbohydrates, protein is an inefficient fuel, causing the body to work quite hard to assimilate it and utilize the nutrients in it, which is why high protein diets are so incredibly effective for quick weight loss. The body kicks into high gear and burns tremendous amounts of its resources to break down the density of protein-rich foods. It sounds great, but it's only a quick fix for weight loss. The reality of the situation is that protein, in large quantities, can have negative long-term effects on our health, not to mention our skin.

The effect of excess protein consumption and the resulting toxic waste buildup shows itself quite dramatically on the skin. The blood feeds the delicate cells, so the quality of that blood is essential to healthy, vital skin. It only stands to reason then, that when our blood grows toxic from waste buildup in the body, our skin will suffer the consequences. Skin, like the delicate leaves of a plant, begins to wither and die, growing tough and leatherlike, prone to wrinkles and premature aging and dryness. As animal protein and fat harden in the body, a layer of saturated fat builds up under the surface of the skin, clogging the pores, inhibiting waste release and blocking moisture intake. As a result, the skin hardens and wrinkles, not unlike a desert floor, cracking open, starved for moisture. And since this toxic buildup of fat and waste is not uniform in its accumulation, the skin will also take on an uneven texture, splotchy color, thickening, pimples, and even callouses.

The downside of excessive protein consumption can have an even darker side, affecting the health of our bones. As excess amounts of protein are consumed, more calcium is leached from the bones. The more calcium we lose to this process, the thinner and weaker our bones become, and the risk of osteoporosis becomes a real threat. In a culture where we consume so much protein, we are plagued by calcium deficiencies—supplementing our diet with more and more milligrams of precious calcium. Studies have shown that women consuming a diet that leans more toward plant food, rather than animal food (not necessarily vegetarian), show far less occurrences of bone degeneration than their sisters consuming more protein. Ironically, as simplistic as it sounds, if we would simply cut back our intake of dense protein, we wouldn't require calcium supplementing on such an obsessive scale. Our bodies would make a natural balance and our bones would be healthy for our entire lifetime. We would stand tall and strong, with elegant spines, soft, supple skin, and a vital glow.

A WORD ABOUT SMOKING

While smoking is not really diet related, this habit wreaks havoc on the skin (not to mention the lungs). Laced with chemicals, cigarettes overwork and tax the liver, gallbladder, kidneys, lungs, and large intestines to the breaking point, which shows itself on the skin as splotchy color, broken capillaries just under the surface of the skin, puffiness under the eyes, and overall redness or a yellowish cast. Coupled with premature aging from the overworked organ systems and the drying effects of hot smoke, cigarettes create the skin of our nightmares, making us slaves to moisturizers, foundations, and concealers, as this lethal habit robs our skin of moisture, vitality, and youth.

Glow Is More Than Skin-Deep

As we have seen here, food influences our skin quite strongly by the energy that it creates in our organs and systems. With the skin receiving about one third of the blood supply in the body, the nourishment that gets to the skin is vital to its health and appearance. The condition of the skin—from the epidermis to the dermis, to the sebum to the connective tissue—depends completely on the quality of nutrients fed it by the blood. Our skin reflects the condition of various organs and systems of the body, making it vital to its health and appearance that we understand our internal environment and how it shows on our face.

In looking at your skin to determine its health, focus on three characteristics: color, condition, and marks appearing on the skin. A glowing complexion is one that is uniform in color and texture, free of bumps and lumps, pimples, lines, spots, or dots. (Even though we can keep them at bay a bit longer with healthy food choices, wrinkles are inevitable.)

OUR SKIN'S CONDITION AND CONSTITUTION

Just like the rest of the body, we must differentiate between our skin's constitution and condition before we can look at ourselves and judge our health. Normal, healthy skin should be clear, smooth, slightly shiny, and ever so slightly moist to the touch. It should feel supple and lush, smooth and lusty. It should beg to be touched, irresistible, glowing. If our internal environment grows unbalanced, it will show on our skin.

As in all disorders of the body, the basic causes of our discomfort and symptoms of illness are caused by our daily diet and life choices. While other factors will always contribute to our troubles, food is at the root of our glowing health or lack of it. In our modern application of beauty treatments, we work externally only, and our endless efforts often yield results that are less than satisfying. We labor so hard on the outside, ignoring the inside. However, natural, beautiful, glowing skin develops easily as a result of a naturally balanced diet.

We are born with perfect skin. Think about how many times we have run our hands enviably over a baby's bottom, wondering what happened to our own skin. That skin, that perfect, soft, flawless skin was the constitutional condition of our skin. The ravages of time and environment, of course, take a toll. Exposure to the harshness of pollution and weather will toughen our skin, compromising the softness that was ours at birth. Trouble arises when, on top of the environmental beating, we overwork our body's organ systems, wearing us down, leaving us with tired, wrinkled, loose skin, as well as any number of complexion woes.

Wet Skin: Characterized most often by sweaty palms, wet skin can be an overall condition, especially evident on the face. While healthy skin will be slightly moist, wet skin is another condition altogether, showing as perpetually wet skin, excessive sweating, and breakouts.

Wet skin is indicative of thinner blood, rapid metabolism and pulse, as well as excessive perspiration and urination. This condition affects more than the look of our skin, it is usually accompanied by diarrhea, fatigue, foggy thinking, forgetfulness, thinning hair, and all sorts of aches and pains in the ears, teeth, and gums. Caused by excessive consumption of water-producing foods such as fruit; juices; soft drinks; too much liquid in general; soft dairy, like milk and yogurt; sugar; and soft, watery sweets. All of these foods produce water in the body in an attempt to stabilize the extreme nature of what we are choosing to eat.

Cravings for these foods are directly proportionate to our consumption of salt, protein, and carbohydrates as the body strives for its equilibrium. As we consume dense foods like strong salts and animal proteins or simple carbohydrates, our body will begin to seek moisture to "cool" our internal environment and to aid in the smoother assimilation of these foods. To satisfy the need for more moisture, we begin to crave soft, creamy foods, sweets, and liquids.

To balance the fluid in the body, a comprehensive approach to balanced eating must be established. Our skin's moisture will quickly be restored to proper balance when our diet reflects a moderate intake of all flavors and textures.

Oily Skin: How many products have we all purchased to blot the excess oil oozing from our pores, most notably in the "T-Zone"—the forehead, nose, and chin? While normal skin will be slightly moist, oily skin is indicative of another condition of excess and is characterized by not only the oil on the skin but enlarged pores and puffiness.

Oily skin is an indication that the liver, gallbladder, and pancreas are not functioning properly, most likely due to excesses in our diet. The lungs and kidneys are also growing sluggish due to overwork. Oily skin shows us that congestion is forming in various organs, inhibiting their efficient function, as well as the possible formation of gall and kidney stones.

Caused by the excessive consumption of fat in the diet, or by a disorder in fat metabolism, oily skin is easily remedied with changes in our daily food choices. Lowering our intake of fatty foods; protein, animal and vegetable; starchy carbohydrates like white flour, white bread, and white pasta; eggs; sugar; and even vegetable oils will quickly alleviate the symptoms of oily skin.

An interesting point about oily skin is that no matter what you choose to eat, overeating, even the healthiest foods, will aggravate the condition. Smaller portions of food will help the condition to clear more quickly. Reduction in the size of pores will take a longer period of time to change, but you will find almost immediate improvements in the texture of your skin with a few moderate diet changes. No more blotting!

Dry Skin: This is one of the most interesting skin conditions. Its cause is either dehydration or the excessive consumption of fats and oils. While that may seem paradoxical, it's not. The tightness, flakes, and even itchiness we associate with dry skin are indicators that there is a relatively large amount of fat and cholesterol in our diet.

Dry skin is often caused by the accumulation of layers of fat under the surface of the skin, which prevents the skin from absorbing moisture and from releasing toxins. With the skin unable to absorb moisture, it grows dry and dehydrated. Our first response is to either eat more fat and oil, or to apply oily moisturizers to the surface of the skin. Both of these methods will simply perpetuate the accumulation of fat under the skin and our dry skin will continue to plague us. Even minor cases of dry skin, like flaky shins in the winter or our face feeling tight after washing, are indicators that our internal environment is under siege.

Along with the aggravation of tight, dry skin, other conditions will most likely exist as a result of the hardening of the fat under the skin. Irregular heartbeat, hardening of the arteries, accumulation of hard fat around the liver, gallbladder, lungs, large intestines, spleen, and pancreas, as well as tight, hard muscles, are most often present with dry skin.

An extreme condition, the best way to alleviate the symptoms is to eliminate (or at least minimize) extreme foods such as meat, eggs, poultry, and dairy foods, as well as sugary sweets. Adding moisture to the diet with whole grains, vegetables, and beans will have your skin soft and moist in a few months.

Rough Skin: Rough or coarse skin is another extreme skin condition and is, not surprisingly, caused by extreme dietary habits. Its cause is excessive consumption of dense proteins and fats and is often accompanied by splotchy coloring or white patches on the skin. On the other end of the spectrum, excessive consumption of fruit, juices, sugary sweets, soft drinks, or chemicals can also cause this condition. This rough skin condition is often accompanied by a slight red color. When caused by protein and saturated fats, rough skin is more difficult to change and will take more time to see results.

Caused by the accumulation of hard fat in the liver and kidneys, this condition is most often accompanied by hardening of the arteries. With this condition of the skin, you will probably also see other symptoms, including stiffness in the neck and shoulders, pain in the joints, general fatigue, frequent intestinal upset, and rigid thinking. When rough skin is caused by overconsumption of sweets and chemicals, it will change very quickly. Along with enlarged pores and sweat glands, other symptoms of the condition include irregular pulse, excessive perspiration, a racing heart, vertigo, an excessively sensitive nature, and frequent emotional upsets. Caused by disorders in the circulatory and nervous symptoms, this condition is quite sensitive and can be altered easily.

In both cases of rough skin, a balanced diet is the key to restoring our skin to its normal soft, smooth texture. Reduction, or elimination, of extreme foods will allow the body to regain its internal balance, which will be reflected in our flawless, smooth complexion.

Loose Skin: Flabby or doughy skin is a very common condition in people today, and it's really no surprise. Characterized by skin that looks washed out, with little or no elasticity, doughy skin can appear anywhere on the body, but is most often found on the face, chest, and abdomen. Caused by excessive consumption of dairy foods, sugar, and white flour, this condition can be changed with dietary modifications. Loose skin is an indication that congestion is accumulating in many places in the body, including the sinus cavities, inner ear, breast tissue, lungs, liver, gallbladder, kidneys, and various glands. Within this condition, we may also see symptoms like hay fever, hearing problems, chronic coughing, spitting mucus, gall and kidney stones, and vaginal discharge, along with laziness, fatigue, and foggy thinking.

A more balanced eating plan, rich in the fiber of whole grains and vegetables, with a reduction in animal foods and simple sugar but with a sensible amount of vegetable quality fat included, will help to restore the skin to its normal state of firmness.

Wrinkles

Oh, those little lines and creases . . . We hate them and struggle with products, potions, lotions, peels, and surgeries to rid our faces of the inevitable tracks of experience. While we can't prevent them infinitely, we can delay their occurrence.

Wrinkles on our faces begin on the inside. Poor digestion and sluggish circulation prevent both nutrients and energy from properly nourishing the skin, thereby weakening it. As it weakens, it wrinkles and sags.

A diet rich in saturated fats, protein, and salt, as well as sweets and sugars, will leave the skin depleted of vital nutrients, while our clogged veins and arteries struggle to feed our starving skin.

To prevent, minimize, and even reduce the appearance of wrinkles, the answer is simple—vitamin C. Vitamin C, which maintains the production of collagen, the connective tissue that holds skin in place, is your best bet for maintaining a youthful, line-free face. While you can supplement with vitamin C, the best sources for this essential nutrient include dark leafy greens, like kale, collards, and broccoli, lemons, green tea, oranges, and tangerines. Using these foods regularly in cooking will help a great deal in keeping your skin as young as you feel.

Pimples

Perfect, flawless, glowing skin, free of acne and pimples, is not just a dream. Clear, beautiful skin is simply the result of a natural, balanced diet.

There are numerous glands in the body responsible for the production of oil, but they are most plentiful in the areas of the face, back, and chest, with as many as five thousand glands per square inch of skin. When the body falls into a state of imbalance, the sebum secreted by these glands becomes excessive and abnormal. Pimples are visible signs that there is an imbalance in the body, representing the elimination of excess, toxic waste. When the buildup is more than the body can process through elimination organs, the skin jumps into the fray, ridding itself of excess through our oil-producing glands and pores.

In normal, balanced skin, the oil produced in the sebaceous glands of the skin flows through the pores, taking dead skin cells that flake off the inside of the skin follicle with it. If the production of oil is excessive, the flow is inhibited, causing the dead skin cells to clump, forming a plug that blocks the flow of oil to the surface of the skin. Eventually, the dead skin cells, oil, and naturally occurring bacteria from the base of the gland clump together and completely block the pore opening. The pore expands to discharge the toxic buildup, forming a tiny, swollen bump, the birth of a pimple.

Blackheads form as bacteria, dead cells, and oil continue to multiply, and the pore is stretched, allowing air to enter. The darkened spot, or blackhead, is not accumulated dirt, but is in fact melanin, a skin pigment that darkens when exposed to air and light. No matter how many pore-cleansing strips you apply, until you stop the buildup of dead cells in the pores, you'll never be rid of blackheads.

If the condition of buildup continues unchecked, pressure increases in the follicle, breaking through the oil gland walls and spilling into the dermis. Blood capillaries expand and white cells jump into action, gathering in the affected area to ward off trouble. The result of all this activity is redness, swelling, and irritation, the beginning of full-blown acne.

Caused by a diet of extremes, particularly animal protein and fat, acne is strongly influenced by androgens, including testosterone, which causes a contracting and accumulating effect in the bloodstream, causing fatty acids to build up around the sebaceous glands, where they turn into sebum and are discharged by the body through the pores. In short, combining strongly contractive animal foods with the stepped-up production of testosterone that comes with puberty creates the perfect recipe for teenage acne. While undesirable, acne is actually a natural self-defense mechanism that the body uses to aid in the discharge of excess, in its attempt to balance an extreme condition. The result of an imbalanced diet, acne is a condition that no one need suffer from. By simply changing the way we eat, with our diet centering on whole grains, vegetables, and beans, we will see dramatic improvements in this condition. It will take time, but a balanced eating plan will yield long-term results, without the serious risk of side effects from strong antibiotics and other drugs commonly used to treat the symptoms.

The Message from Our Pimples

While not a welcome sight, pimples reveal information about our condition and should have our full attention. In general, pimples are expansive in nature, even when caused by the contracting effects of dense animal fats. Simply the body's attempt to discharge fat, rather than minerals and other excesses, pimples are more than just inconvenient and unattractive. Pimples affect more than just our skin. They are a revelation of deeper accumulations of excess fat and actually aid the body in ridding itself of toxic buildup.

The location of our pimples reveals to us which organs are being overwhelmed by fat buildup, so we know how to adjust our eating. Here's the message from those little bumps. (For those on the face, see pages 31–38.) If pimples appear on the shoulders, the digestive tract suffers from fat accumulation, while blemishes on the chest and/or upper back show that the heart and lungs are working very hard to discharge accumulated fat buildup.

It's easy to see that pimples mean more to us than unattractive skin—they are a reflection of our health. Switching to a more natural, whole way of eating will result in very few (if any) breakouts, with pimples arising to signal a minor imbalance and disappearing as quickly as balance is restored.

Freckles and Other Cute Spots

Growing up, I thought that being a redhead was the cause for the freckles that were generously sprinkled over my nose, cheeks, arms, hands, and shoulders. My lifestyle has revealed to me that I was wrong. Although considered cute as a child, freckles were the plague of my youth and no amount of makeup would cover the sea of brown dots that covered me. If only I had known that my ancestry had less to do with the freckles than I thought, I could have had relief much sooner.

Generally appearing on the more peripheral, expansive areas of the body—the face, cheeks, arms, shoulders, and hands—freckles are caused as the body tries to eliminate excessive accumulation of simple carbohydrates in the body, including refined sugar, honey, fruit and fruit juices, and milk sugar. Expansive by nature (the result of sugars), freckles will rise to the surface of the skin, especially during the summer, when the contractive nature of the sun attracts the expansive nature of the freckles.

Produced by melanin, freckles are caused by diet and environment. Melanin is formed by melanocytes, the branch-shaped part of the cells found in the lowest part of the epidermis. While all people have just about the same amount of these cells, diet and environment influence the amount of melanin they produce, which in turn, determine the pigmentation of the skin. The excessive consumption of dense fats blocks the skin, causing erratic production of melanin, resulting in uneven, speckled pigmentation—freckles.

Age spots are different than freckles, in look and in cause. Larger than freckles and flat, age spots usually show up on the hands, face, and upper chest and are the direct result of excessive consumption of simple carbohydrates, refined sugar, honey, and tropical fruits. As accumulating sugars gather at the surface of the skin (so the body can eliminate them), they stimulate concentrated production of melanin and can create the large, unattractive spots we call age spots. And while these spots can appear at any age, they seem to be the plague of old age, as the body responds to years and years of sugar consumption.

Both freckles and age spots are the result of extremes in the diet and can fade or even disappear when the diet is refurbished to be more balanced, centered on whole grains, seasonal vegetables, and beans. I continue to be surprised, to this day, at the smooth, freckle-free skin that I now enjoy.

Moles and Other Bumps and Lumps

Like other abnormalities on our skin, moles or other growths on our skin are a form of discharge of accumulated excess. Moles, warts, and other bumps have specific causes and need not be a scourge on our perfect skin.

Moles come in a variety of colors and textures, from bluish-black to brown or flesh-colored and from smooth and flat to rough and hairy, but are caused by the excessive consumption of protein or by chronic overeating, particularly of dense fats. With this as the cause, in Asia, moles were said to form on egocentric people prone to indulgence. With proper, balanced eating, moles can fade, reduce, and even drop off the skin.

And then there's warts. Like other growths on the skin, warts are caused by the excessive accumulation of protein, but in the case of warts, the protein is specific. The excessive consumption of milk and other dairy products, coupled with large quantities of simple sugars in the diet, warts tend to appear in people who consume a lot of sugar and fat together. Ice cream, milk chocolate, yogurt, and the like may taste great but can cause lumps and bumps on the skin.

Even in the case where warts are caused by viruses, it's important to remember that a virus's ability to trigger the abnormal discharge of fat and sugar through the skin is largely influenced by the food choices of the person. We just can't escape the responsibility of what goes into our mouth.

While warts can be treated symptomatically, in order to rid yourself of them for good, a diet shift must occur. Elimination of the foods responsible for their formation is the key, as well as diet adjustments that help the body to break down and efficiently discharge the accumulated fats. Use of grains like barley, and vegetables like daikon and shiitake mushrooms can be quite helpful in ridding our skin of warts, as well as preventing the chronic formation of them.

Oh, Baby, Those Beauty Marks

Black or dark-brown spots, usually flat to the skin, are known as "beauty marks" and are quite different from moles and warts, both in character and in cause. Appearing on specific areas of the face, beauty marks are caused by internal conditions. Moles, freckles, and warts appear as the result of external heat and light, while beauty marks are caused by an internal heat. Beauty marks most often appear after the occurrence of a high fever, as in the case of pneumonia, rheumatic fever, kidney, or bladder infections. The beauty mark will appear on the face or body in the area that reflects the condition of the organ or system most affected by the disease or fever.

In both Asian healing arts and Italian folklore, "beauty marks" are said to be a sign that someone loves you very much.

You're So Vein

Varicose veins, the plague of leg beauty, occurs when the surface veins in the legs become blocked with accumulated fat, causing them to swell and bulge.

Caused primarily by the excessive consumption of extreme expansive foods, varicose veins are often painful and always unsightly. Fluids, milk, fruit juice, black tea, coffee, sugar-laced drinks, coupled with dense fats, especially butter, cream, cheese, and eggs, are the primary cause of the blockage that causes the swollen, bulging veins that we know as varicose veins.

While consuming a healthy, balanced diet can prevent varicose veins, once the veins are damaged and swollen, the best you can hope for is a reduction of their appearance. They won't completely disappear, but they will diminish and the pain will be greatly reduced as circulation is restored.

Along with a proper diet, a specific topical application can bring some relief. Applying alternately hot and cold towels to the affected veins for ten minutes before bed can be very helpful in diminishing appearance and symptoms of varicose veins.

As we have seen here, our skin is more than just the covering of the body that holds our bits in place. The most peripheral organ system, our skin strongly reflects our strengths and weaknesses. Perfect, supple, irresistible, touchable skin is ours for the taking. Responsibility for what we consume, smart food choices, and sensible skin care result in skin that begs to be touched.

Glowingly Expressive Hands and Feet

Your Hands

Our hands are lovely, expressive appendages of communication, work, art, craft, and creation. Do you have soft, supple, well-formed hands—hands of sonnets and poetry? Or when you look down, do you see cracked, irritated skin, ragged nails, split fingertips, gnarled knuckles?

Our hands and our feet tell a great deal about us and are a fascinating, lifelong study in diagnosis. We associate palm reading with psychics and fortune-telling, but our hands reveal more about us than whether we'll marry or not. In traditional healing arts, the hands and feet are considered to be conductors of energy, both into and out of, the body. As end points for our meridiens (the energy pathways that run through the body, creating life as we know it), our hands and feet reveal a great deal about the health and function of various organ systems, our emotional well-being, and yes, even our future tendencies, based on what is revealed in our palms.

For purposes of diagnosis, the hand is divided into two areas, the palm and the fingers, with each revealing specific characteristics. The palm is reflective of our physical constitution, while the fingers show more of our emotional and mental tendencies. For purposes of seeing your own health, there is a simple guideline to use. Many people show distinct differences in both hands, particularly on the palms. To see your physical tendencies, look at the dominant hand, the hand you favor for use. To see your potential, as well as spiritual tendencies, look at the other hand.

The arms, hands, and fingers (as well as the legs, feet, and toes), grew outward from the body as organs were developing internally. The result is that the hands and fingers reflect specific organs and their functions.

The thumb, down to its base, reflects the health and function of the lungs. Our first finger, down to its base and continuing along the same region of the palm and back of the hand, reflects the health and function of the large intestine. The second finger, down to its base and continuing along the corresponding regions of the palm and the back of the hand, to the center of the hand, reflects the health and function of the center of the body, the heart, stomach, abdominal region, as well as the circulatory and reproductive systems. The third finger, down to its base and continuing along the corresponding regions of the palm and the back of the hand, controls our very vitality, along with internal temperature and energy flow within the body. Our smallest finger, the pinky, has many jobs. Our smallest finger, down to its base and continuing along the palm side, reflects the health and function of the heart and circulatory systems, while on the back of the hand, it reflects the health and function of the small intestine.

This information is important to us, as we can now see how conditions of the fingers, accidents, and abnormalities are created by the condition of various organs. For example, if we are working in the kitchen and cut or burn a specific finger, it shows that the corresponding organ is out of balance that day and has called our attention to the situation.

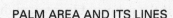

PALM AREA AND ITS LINES

a. Lifeline

b. Head or intellect line

c. Love or emotion line

THE LINES OF YOUR PALM

On the palm side of the hand, we divide it into three sections, based on the three major lines of the hand. Beginning with our lifeline, running from the root of the thumb to the base of the palm, we see the health and condition of the digestive and respiratory systems. We call this line the lifeline, because the organ health it reflects is vital to our very existence.

Our head line, or line of intellect, runs across the center of the palm, from the thumb across to the pinky-finger side. Reflective of the health and function of our nervous system, this line shows the function of our brain and nervous reactions.

Our love line, or the line of emotion, running across the palm, at the base of the fingers, beginning between the first and second fingers and crossing to the pinky-finger side of the palm, is said to reflect the health and function of our circulatory and excretory systems. We call this the line of emotion, because the function of our blood, lymph, and urinary organs has a powerful impact on our emotional well-being.

The other lines showing on the palm mean different things in different cultures. One characteristic remains constant, however. The more lines showing on your palm, the more complex and layered is your personality. A palm that shows fewer lines shows a simple, straightforward character.

As with the rest of our bodies, our hands have a constitutional character and they show the condition that we create. It's interesting to see how our inherent character is reflected in the constitutional character of our hands, showing our natural tendencies.

THE SHAPE OF YOUR PALM

Looking at your hand, if the palm is longer than the fingers, this shows a strong constitution, with a persevering character and great strength. If the palm and fingers are the same length, this shows a constitution oriented toward more mental activities and a tendency to be more physically delicate. If the palm is shorter than the fingers, this shows a spiritual orientation, with a very delicate physical character, with little resistance.

A thicker palm is indicative of a sound and healthy constitution, with the potential for a long, healthy, and active life. A thinner palm indicates a more delicate constitution, representing less vitality and more struggles in life.

A wide palm is the result of being nourished by a balanced diet and shows physical strength and good vitality, while a narrow palm is the result of a diet rich in sugar and other sweets and shows a more delicate constitution.

THE COLOR OF YOUR PALM

Take a look at your palm. Do you see clear, uniform color that matches the rest of you? Or is the skin on the palm irregular or splotchy? Is your palm wet, dry, or supple to the touch? Are there areas of the palm that are sensitive to touch, even painful? All of these symptoms indicate specific imbalances in your health.

A normal, healthy palm is uniform and clear in color, with soft, supple skin, and is free of swelling and pain.

If the overall color of the palm is reddish, this indicates that the heart and circulatory system are aggravated and overworked, due to the excessive consumption of stimulants in the diet; hot spices, caffeine, alcohol, and simple sugar are most often the cause of this color change.

If a purple color develops, particularly in the area of the palm that runs from the little finger to the base of the palm, it indicates sluggish function of both the circulatory and excretory systems, resulting from the excessive intake of extremes in the diet, from saturated fats to simple sugars to stimulants.

Should the palm reflect a yellowish color, this indicates that liver, gallbladder, excretory and circulatory systems are clogged and sluggish. Caused by the excessive consumption of saturated animal fats, particularly eggs, meat, and cheese, this condition may also be the result of too much oil and fat in the diet, without enough exercise to help circulate these fats through the system. Interestingly, we often see this condition in people who consume large quantities of carrots and carrot juice, winter squash and pumpkin, indicating a buildup of beta carotene in the system, much less harmful than the buildup of saturated fats.

Looking at the very center of the palm, you should note a slight indentation. If pressure is applied, this area shows good health if it is soft and pain-free. If this region of the palm is rigid and there is slight pain with pressure, it indicates that you are overtired, resulting in sluggish digestion. Regardless of diet, if proper rest doesn't balance our activity and lifestyle, this condition will develop.

If the color of the center of the palm matches the rest of the palm, it shows overall good health. Should this area grow red, the circulatory system is aggravated from the excessive intake of stimulants. Purple color shows that respiration and reproductive function grow sluggish from the struggle to balance extremes in the diet. A yellow color develops when the liver and gallbladder are overcome by our intake of saturated fats. I make the distinction between the center of the palm and the rest of the palm, because on many occasions, the color of the center of the palm differs greatly from the rest of the hand. Since this region of the palm shows our overall vitality, the imbalances in our body show here before the rest of the palm.

Now look at the root of the thumb, the fleshy mound (sometimes called the Mound of Venus) just below the thumb itself. This area of the palm shows health when it matches the color of the rest of the palm. Should the color change, imbalance is indicated. If the mound changes to reflect a purple, blue, or reddish color, it indicates that digestion is in disorder. The large and small intestines' functions are growing sluggish due to dietary imbalance. Specifically, this coloring shows that the intestines are clogged with accumulated fats, saturated and unsaturated, dairy foods, and refined flour products, all of which greatly inhibit the function of the digestive system. If you look on the back of the hand and a similar color is reflected at the root of the thumb, the condition is more pronounced in the large intestine.

Since you're looking at the back of your hand, let's continue here. While good health shows as uniform color, normal hands will react to weather and environment, turning red or purple in cold or extreme heat. Should these colors arise at any other time, however, it indicates imbalances in the circulatory, excretory, digestive, and nervous systems, due to the excessive consumption of expansive foods, particularly artificial chemicals, drugs, and medications. You will see this condition, to a lesser degree, in people who consume large quantities of simple sugars, processed foods, and who take large numbers of vitamins. However, like the palm, a healthy hand is clear, smooth, and uniform in color, matching the rest of you.

THE SKIN OF YOUR HANDS

The skin of the hand, like the skin on the rest of the body, reflects health when it is smooth, clear, and free of abnormalities.

Like the rest of the skin on the body, the skin on the hands is fed by the nutrients we choose daily. Abnormalities in the skin of our hands show that the heart, kidneys, and reproductive organs are in disorder. Dry, wet, oily, rough, chafed, split or peeling, the skin on our hands reflects the core of our vitality.

Dry skin on the hands, or skin that splits, peels, chafes, or roughens, is the result of excessive consumption of saturated fats, which are accumulating around the kidneys, around the heart and in the reproductive system. While minor versions of dry skin can be caused by the excessive intake of simple sugars and stimulants, as well as chemicals, dry skin on the hands is not the result of hard work or dishwater. If saturated fat builds up under the skin, as well as around the kidneys, dry skin will result. Fat under the skin prevents the discharge of waste and the absorption of moisture, while accumulating fat inhibits the kidneys in their job of discharging toxins from the body. Like other dry skin, the more lotion we slather over our hands, the more blocked the skin and the more dry the skin. To alleviate symptoms of dry skin, while altering eating patterns, look for a light, not-oil-based moisturizer that will not clog the pores.

Externally, the only cause of dry skin on the hands would be the use of chemicals in your work, like paint, paint thinners, and other chemical solvents, and other than a job change, is difficult to heal and must be dealt with topically.

Excessively moist or oily skin on the hands results from consuming large amounts of simple sugars in our diet. Quickly turning to fat in various organs, simple sugars overwhelm our discharge organs, leaving the job of ridding the body of excess fats to the skin, resulting in wet or oily skin on the hands.

STRONG, FLEXIBLE HANDS

The joints in our hands, wrists, and fingers show both our physical and mental flexibility. If the hands, fingers, and wrists are supple and mobile, it shows that we are physically flexible and emotionally stable, while rigidity in these joints shows that our body is growing hard and our emotions are rigid.

To maintain an adaptable life, to balance with grace, all of the little road blocks that are thrown in our path, it's important to maintain a flexible body. The greater the flexibility in the hands, fingers, and wrists, the greater our capacity to adapt in life, to changes in our environment, in our life patterns, in our bodies. Flexibility in this area of the body indicates that our muscles, arteries, and nervous system are supple, smooth, and efficiently functioning to carry us through life.

Rigidity of the fingers, wrists, and hands are the result of the excessive consumption of animal foods. A diet rich in saturated fats, protein, and cholesterol will overwork and exhaust the body, as well as result in hard, rigid muscles, swollen knuckles and joints, clogged, hardened arteries, and sluggish nervous function. With this rigidity of the hands, fingers, and joints, we most often also see a stubborn will, with little inclination to embrace change.

YOUR FINGERS

For purposes of seeing your health, we'll divide the fingers into three sections, the base area, closest to the palm, the mid-section, and the tip.

The bases of the fingers reflect the health and function of our digestive and respiratory systems, with the mid-sections reflecting the health and function of our nervous system and the tips showing the health and function of our circulatory and excretory functions. This is important to note, as conditions and colors of the skin on the fingers will indicate various conditions. For instance, if redness occurs on any particular section of the finger, the corresponding organs and systems are aggravated and overworked. Should the skin on any section of the fingers grow dry, the corresponding organ is accumulating saturated fats, while pimples or white spots on the fingers show an accumulation of simple sugars and soft fat in the systems that correspond to that section of the fingers.

Look at your fingers. When stretched out, they should look relatively straight and generally balanced in structure. Stretched to their full length, under normal, healthy conditions, the second finger is the longest, the first finger is second, the third finger is third in length, and of course, the pinky finger is shortest, with the thumb set lowest on the hand, with its tip lower than all the other fingers.

Remembering that the fingers correspond to different organs and their functions, the thumb to the lungs, the first finger to the large intestine, the second finger to the circulatory system, the third to stomach and overall vitality, and the pinky to the heart and small intestine, different conditions of the fingers will mean different things to our condition.

Looking at your fingers, if the first finger is longer than the second finger, it illustrates a tendency toward weakness in the large intestine, as this longer finger shows a naturally expanded condition of this organ system. If the third finger is taller than the first finger, approaching the height of the second finger, it shows a tendency toward a weaker stomach and resulting vitality, while an abnormally long pinky finger shows the tendency toward chronic heart and small intestine disorders.

Your Fingertips

Take a look at your fingertips. Their shape gives you some insight into your natural tendencies and character, based on your constitution. Squarish fingertips are the result of physically robust parents and a diet of stronger foods being eaten during pregnancy, creating a person who tends to be physically active, determined, and aggressive.

Rounder fingertips are the result of healthy parents, with a nutritionally balanced diet being eaten during pregnancy. Plenty of stronger and lighter foods in the diets creates a person who is active, energetic, and generally positive in their outlook.

Narrow, more pointed fingertips are the result of more delicate parentage, less physically active, the result of a diet oriented more toward raw vegetables, fruits, juices, sweets and sugars, with fewer strong foods being consumed. This kind of diet creates a more delicate constitution, with a sensitive, artistic nature and an interest in the arts and spiritual pursuits.

Swollen fingertips are not the result of our constitutional tendencies but rather are created by our diet choices. This condition of the fingertips is caused by extremes in the diet, as our bodies struggle on the roller coaster between simple sugars, alcohol, and caffeine and saturated fats, protein, and salt. Not only taxing on our health, this style of eating makes for a self-centered, aggressive, and negative personality.

Conditions of the Fingers

The fingers and fingertips are considered to be additional exit points for excess energy and nutrients and, as such, will take on certain conditions and symptoms based on our internal health and balance.

If, on waking, your fingers are usually swollen, you need to look at your intake of simple sugars, which are not only depleting the blood of minerals, but are inhibiting both the kidneys and large intestine in their ability to regulate moisture, leaving you bloated and swollen. With this condition, we often see a tendency toward anxiety and depression.

Cracking, splitting skin on the fingers, especially at the tips, again is indicative that your diet is a bit too rich in sweet things and needs more balance. Also the result of drugs, chemicals, and medications, this condition of the fingers shows that the circulatory and reproductive systems are weakening. If unchecked, this condition can result in loss of interest in passion and romance, along with an overall sense of fatigue.

White, fatty deposits around the fingertips show that fat is accumulating in the body. Caused by the excessive consumption of animal fats, proteins, and dairy products, as well as too much vegetable fat, this condition shows that the lymph system is clogged and sluggish and kidney and liver function is overwhelmed and growing weak. Along with this condition, we often see an anxious, fearful, impatient nature.

If the fingers take on a purplish cast, particularly near the tips, it shows that the lungs and overall respiratory function are weakening due to the excessive consumption of expansive foods, in particular, caffeine, simple sugars, and stimulating hot spices. Along with this condition of the fingers, we often see an overly sensitive and nervous nature, as well as chronically cold hands and feet.

Hard, dry, flaky skin on the fingers, particularly around the tips, shows that dairy products and animal protein and fat in the diet, especially eggs, are causing hardening of the arteries and stiffness of the muscles. Along with this condition of the fingers, we often see rigid and narrow thinking.

If the skin on the fingers is overly soft, mushy, and peels easily, it shows that more liquid than we need is in our diet, but in particular, soft drinks, fruit juices, alcohol, and other stimulating beverages. This condition of the fingers is indicative of overactive heart and circulatory function, weakening both and creating an overly sensitive and emotionally volatile nature.

If the skin on the palm side of the fingertips looks shriveled and wrinkled, as though you have been in a bath for too long or swimming for an extended period of time, this indicates that there are not enough minerals in your bloodstream. This condition is caused by the excessive consumption of simple sugars that leach minerals from the blood, the inability to assimilate minerals in our foods, or simply from a lack of minerals in the foods we choose to eat and is easily remedied by diet changes.

AND NOW FOR SOMETHING COMPLETELY DIFFERENT

Now that we've talked about seeing our health in our hands, let's have a bit of fun. We've all seen palm readers and fortune-tellers at the ready to reveal our future. Whether you embrace that as truth or debunk it as entertainment, it's interesting to see what ancient cultures say is revealed in your hands and fingers.

With no scientific facts or studies to back this up, you may be surprised at the accuracy of these next observations of the hands.

Stretch out your fingers and look at your hand, palm down. With the fingers stretched taut and kept together, do you see spaces between your fingers or are they tight, snugly fitting together? In the case of spaces between your fingers, it is said, this shows a person who loves to spend money; it slips through your fingers, so to speak. Tight, snugly fitting fingers, on the other hand, show a person who saves for a rainy day and spends wisely. This is the person to be in charge of the checkbook.

Keep your fingers stretched out, again, palm down. Each finger is said to represent specific people. The thumb represents our parents; the first finger shows our family; the second finger shows you; the third finger reflects our friends, with the pinky finger showing our children (whether we have them or not). Look at how the other fingers orient to the second finger, the one representing you. Does your first finger lean slightly toward the second? That shows, it is said, that family members tend to lean on you. Perhaps you're the family peacekeeper.

How about the third finger? Does it lean toward the second? That indicates that your friends are likely to come to you for help, assistance, and support. Your nurturing personality makes you a compassionate shoulder to lean on. If the pinky finger leans in toward the second finger, it shows that your children are also dependent upon you for support and nurturing. Should all three fingers lean in to the second finger, it shows that all in your circle of family and friends count on you to be a pillar of strength and support.

On the other hand, should the first, third, or pinky finger curve away from the second finger, representing you, it means that the corresponding people, family, friends, children are independent and like to stand on their own two feet.

Now take a look at the finger that represents you, the second finger. Is it straight and tall, showing independence? Or does the second finger lean toward the first finger, showing dependence on family, or toward the third, showing that we lean on our friends for support?

Finally, the thumb represents our parents. When you stretch your hand out, does the thumb form a ninety-degree "L", pointing away from the hand, indicating that our parents gladly gave us independence? Or does the thumb point a bit more upwards, forming a "V", showing a tendency to stay closer to our parents?

Take a look and see what's true for you.

Now for some real palm reading. While you most likely won't see your future husband, or wife, you can see your innate tendencies and character. Understand that what you may see on your palm is simply a tendency, the path you are on if there are no changes to your current lifestyle.

As I said earlier, for many people, the palms of each hand look decidedly different. There's a reason. I also said that when diagnosing your health, it's important to study your dominant hand to see your current physical condition, with the other hand representing your spiritual tendencies, and your unrealized potential.

In many of the cases where we see differing palms, we see that the dominant hand lacks definition. The lines of the hand are not distinct and strong. Instead, the lines are more distinct in the submissive hand. This shows a person who has not found their identity yet, has not found their path, their purpose. Very often, you see this distinction in the lines in the hands in younger people, who are still in the process of becoming. You will also see this kind of distinction of lines between the two hands in people not following their passion, or in people who are living their lives as someone's mother, father, sister, brother, husband, or wife, instead of living in their own identity.

Look at your dominant palm. A strong, clear, long lifeline indicates longevity and prosperity in your lifetime. The lifeline shows our aging process beginning above the thumb and winding around the fleshy mound toward the wrist. Breaks in the lifeline indicate difficulties or health struggles at certain times of life: breaks high in the line show struggles early in life, while breaks lower in the lifeline show difficulties arising later in life. Look closely at the lifeline. Should you see a secondary line split off from the lifeline, it indicates that you will take a different path at that point of your life. Look again. Do you see a line running closely beside the lifeline, mirroring its path? This line, known as a ghost line, is said to indicate that you live your life under strong spiritual protection. Perhaps a departed relative or ancestor or simply a guardian angel is watching over you, lucky, lucky you and your charmed life.

Moving up to the line of intellect, running across the palm, this line shows your tendency toward intellectual pursuits, not how smart you are, but how attracted to matters of the mind you might be. A long, deep line is indicative that you are contented to curl up with a good book or study for the sake of study, while a shorter line indicates a person more prone to action. These are people who study a subject just long enough to grasp it and are itching to get on with it. If you notice that the end of the line of intellect (on the side of the pinky finger) branches out into several smaller lines, it indicates that you are a person who is a true multi-tasker, able to study and focus on more than one topic, quite efficiently and contentedly.

Now look at the thumb side of the line of intellect. Do the line of intellect and the lifeline come together, connecting at the end, making a point? If this is the case, it indicates a person who likes to play it safe, taking only calculated risks in life, much preferring serenity to adventure. If, however, there is a space between the two lines, with no connection at the beginning of the lines, you tend to be a person with a more impulsive nature, more willing to take a risk and jump into a situation before knowing all the facts, or the outcome.

The heart or emotion line is said to show how we express our emotions. If the line is deeply curved, moving from between the first two fingers outward to the pinky side of the palm, it is said that your emotions run deep and that generally, you follow your heart, rather than your head. A straighter line, with a more delicate curve, indicates a more sensible approach to life, with your head generally in charge of your heart. Should you see little branches splitting off either end of the emotion line, it is said to show a fickle nature.

Do you see a line running up the center of your palm, cutting through all the other lines? This line, known as the karma or fate line, is said to indicate that you have a strong belief in a higher power. No matter what you might believe that power to be, you are sure that there's someone or something bigger than us out there. It is also said to indicate strong, creative expression.

Now check out the fleshy mound at the base of your thumb, known as the Mound of Venus. If you see lines running across the mound, from the thumb side toward the center of the palm, it is said to indicate that you love to travel, and if there are a lot of lines, you may get to travel as much as you desire. It is also said that these lines show a love of public speaking.

While there are lots and lots of other lines mapping out your tendencies and character traits, this little primer on what our fingers and palms reveal is just the beginning of seeing the true expressive nature of our hands.

Your Feet

We walk on them, stand on them, run on them, cram them into pointy-toed shoes, totter on them in high heels, seal them into work boots, wing tips, and sneakers, and dance on them all night, light as feathers. We soak them, massage them, trim and decorate them with rings and anklets, work them until they ache with fatigue. But what the feet reveal about our health, and their importance to our overall vitality, is sometimes overlooked, as we go through our day, ever reliant on our tender, telling feet.

As major peripheral parts of the body, the feet and toes are representative of our overall condition, revealing the health and function of various organs and systems. Specific conditions of the feet and toes tell us a great deal about what's going on in our internal environment. Balance and imbalance are revealed to us by our feet and their health.

Normal healthy feet, which reflect a balanced condition, are smooth and soft, with uniform color, free of calluses, bumps, corns, dry, flaky skin, warts and other abnormalities specific to the feet. They show toes that gradually decrease in length from the big toe to the pinky, without abnormal bends and crimps in them.

The Character of the Feet

We don't think much about the size of our feet, unless we're buying shoes, but there's more to it. The length and width of the feet is, of course, proportional to the size of the body, but individual constitutions create differences in our individual feet.

The size of our feet is determined in the womb. Larger feet are indicative of sound health in the middle region of the body, meaning that the spleen, pancreas, stomach, liver, gallbladder, and kidneys are active and functioning efficiently. If you have larger feet, it means that these organs are inherently strong.

Smaller feet are indicative of sound health in both the upper and lower regions of the body, meaning that the lungs, large intestine, heart, and small intestine are active and functioning efficiently. With smaller feet, it shows that these organs are constitutionally strong for you.

The height of the feet (from the floor to the top of the foot) varies with the mother's diet choices while the baby is in the womb. Higher, more narrow feet are the result of a diet richer in protein, resulting in a tendency to be more physically active, as the protein gives more inherent strength. Lower, wider feet, the result of a diet more oriented toward carbohydrates and fluids, show a person attracted more to academic pursuits, rather than physical activities.

The arch of the foot is interesting. Higher arches are the result of more contracted muscles, which allow for more active function of the feet. Created by the consumption of a balanced diet, with less fluid and sweets, these kinds of feet are usually the feet of active, athletic people and are essential in athletes, dancers, and sportsmen. Lower arches are the result of more relaxed muscles in the feet, the result of more liquid in the diet. These are the feet of less physically active people who are, instead, in hot pursuit of aesthetic and spiritual interests. These feet are often found in philosophers, writers, musicians, and artists, as well as spiritual leaders.

Flexibility of the ankle joint and the toes is important in determining our health and attitude. With many moving parts, the toes and ankles should be flexible and able to move in many directions without stiffness or pain, showing vascular strength and supple muscles, due to the consumption of an overall balanced diet. A lack of flexibility in these joints shows hardening of the arteries and stiffness of muscles and is the direct result of a diet rich in saturated fats and cholesterol. A secondary cause of this condition is the consumption of salt-cured or smoked meats, like sausages, lunch meats, pastrami, and corned beef, as the salt and saturated fat create a deadly combination for our arteries and muscles. Interestingly, people with more flexible feet are often referred to as "light on their feet" and have a more positive attitude, while people with stiffer, less flexible feet are often rigid in their movements, as well as in their thinking. Think about how much sense this makes; when your feet are comfortable, you are in a better mood. Do I have to remind you about how cranky you get when your feet hurt?

Looking at your foot on the big toe side, does the ball of the foot protrude? A condition that can develop in childhood or adulthood, this protrusion is a sign that the middle organs of the body are hardening in the area of the liver, spleen, stomach, and pancreas due to specific imbalances in the diet, with salt as the culprit here. Salt and fat, salt and protein, salt and carbohydrates, or salt and salt, this condition indicates stiffness in the organs and muscles of the middle body. With this condition, we often see mental rigidity as well, with the attitude that there are two ways to do something, our way or the wrong way. Cutting back on salt and adding small amounts of dissolving vegetables, like daikon and dried shiitake mushrooms to our diet can easily remedy this condition.

Walk in your normal gait, looking at your feet (taking care not to walk into anything). Do they point inward or outward when you walk? A tight base of the spine causes feet that turn out while walking. The result of the consumption of animal foods in greater quantity than vegetable foods, these feet are said to be a sign of a more progressive, outgoing nature. It is said that people with these feet tend to stride confidently into a room, at the ready to be socially active and in charge.

Feet that turn inward, on the other hand, are created by a more relaxed spine, due to the consumption of little or no animal foods, with more focus being placed on vegetables. These feet are said to be a sign of a more introspective, gentle, and quiet character. We see more outward-pointing feet in modern times, because we eat more animal foods than generations past.

A bit of sexist legend for you: In the Asian healing arts, it was said at one time that men who were healthy had feet that were straight or pointed slightly outward when walking, while women who were healthy had feet that were straight or pointed slightly inward when walking.

The Color of the Feet

Like the rest of the body, healthy feet have smooth skin, with uniform color, without splotches or other discolorations. Changes or differences in the color of the feet show specific internal conditions.

Reddish color on the feet, which is rarely all over, but usually at the periphery—toes, sides, and heels—is due to the expansion of capillaries in the feet and is the result of the excessive consumption of expansive foods, including refined sugars, simple sugars, fruit juices, alcohol, caffeine, soft drinks, chemicals, drugs, and medications. This condition shows that the heart and circulatory systems are aggravated and overworked and is often accompanied by rapid pulse, shallow breathing, and overactive kidney and bladder function, resulting in frequent urination. Reddish color on the feet results in loss of clarity in thinking and general fatigue.

A purplish cast to the feet, again more on the periphery than over the entire foot, is a more serious version of the above condition, which generally progresses to this condition if our diet remains unchanged. This condition indicates that circulation, pulse, and breath are racing, with excretory and even reproductive systems in complete disorder. With this condition, we often see heart trouble, as the blood racing through the veins is nutritionally deficient, due to sugar-leaching minerals and vitamins from the bloodstream.

If the peripheral areas of the feet take on a yellowish tint, this indicates that the liver and gallbladder are struggling and growing hard, with their function inhibited, due to the excessive consumption of saturated animal fats, particularly meat, poultry, and eggs. With this condition, we generally see an overall lack of stamina, with a tendency toward impatience and a lack of compassion for others.

If the feet take on an dark color, it indicates that circulation is growing sluggish, as the kidneys and other excretory organs grow clogged with saturated animal fats. This condition can also be the result of excessive consumption of white flour, long-cooked foods, and a diet that lacks freshness. With this condition, we generally see deep fatigue and a tendency toward negative thinking, depression, and anxiety.

If the feet take on an overly pale complexion, this indicates one of two extreme conditions—weak blood, possibly anemia, or constricted blood flow to the feet due to hardening of the arteries. In the case of anemia, the cause is the excessive consumption of sugars that weaken the blood as they leach minerals and vitamins from the bloodstream. With this condition, we see a lack of strength and stamina, someone who tires easily and is not refreshed by rest and tends to shy away from challenges, lacking the strength to rise to the occasion. In the case of hardened arteries, the cause is the accumulation of saturated fat or salts in the veins and arteries, due to the excessive consumption of animal foods or salty foods. With this condition, we often see racing pulse, rapid heartbeat, poor circulation, as well as rigid thinking and a stubborn nature, but again, a lack of stamina and strength. In both cases of excessively pale feet, there is danger of heart trouble.

A greenish tint to the peripheral parts of the feet indicate that the spleen and lymph function, as well as circulatory function, is abnormal and sluggish, due to the accumulation of fat and congestion around various organs. The result of dairy foods, fatty meats, simple sugars, oily foods, and white-flour products, this condition may also be an indication of cyst formation and is often accompanied by mood swings, sluggish erratic energy, and feelings of self-pity.

Your Toes

"This little piggy went to market; this little piggy stayed home; this little piggy had roast beef; this little piggy had none; this little piggy ran, wee, wee, wee all the way home." This little ditty, sung to many babies as we play with their toes, was designed to amuse and delight. But what if I told you that it also stimulated organ function, making the baby more alert and active? It's true. The toes are more than a vehicle for rings and nail polish.

The toes are the final exit point for our meridiens, so each toe and the area of the foot extending from it, represents certain organs and their functions.

The big toe represents major organs and their function, the outside of the toe represents the health and function of the spleen and pancreas, while the inside of the toe represents the liver and its function. The second and third toes represent the health and function of the stomach, while the fourth toe shows the health and function of the gallbladder. The fifth toe shows the health and function of the bladder.

Look down at your feet, at the length and shape of your toes. In normal health, the toes all decrease in length from the big toe to the pinky. The toes in a healthy person are without deep curves and bends and are free of calluses and discoloration.

What we see most often in people today is the second and third toes being longer than the first toe. This condition is indicative of weakened

stomach function and is constitutional, not something that [...]
with day-to-day choices. If we see that we have that inherent wea[...]
however, we can work to support the function of this important orga[...]
so that we can strengthen and nourish its work in our bodies. People
born with these longer toes, if they are not diligent, can easily develop
stomach ulcers.

Curving of the toes indicates abnormal, overactive organ function.
If the big toe curves in toward the second toe, this shows an overactive
spleen and lymph system, while the function of the liver grows sluggish.
Caused by the excessive consumption of fats and oils from both plant
and animal sources, this condition is usually accompanied by a tendency
toward depression and negativity.

If the pinky toe curves abnormally in toward the fourth toe, or even
overlaps the fourth toe, this indicates that the kidneys and bladder are
aggravated and overworked, caused by the excessive consumption of
liquids and sweets. This condition results not only in frequent urination,
but also in feelings of nervousness and anxiety.

If all the toes curve inward or curl excessively, this indicates that the
major organ systems are overworked and aggravated, with our muscles
and arteries hardening and stiffening. Due to extremes in the diet, from
excessive consumption of saturated animal fats and proteins, particularly
chicken and eggs, as well as simple, refined sugars and other sweets, this
condition is generally accompanied by a lack of strength and stamina, as
well as general fatigue.

Oh, Those Calluses

Hard, saturated fats are the cause of many of our health woes, but
we are often unaware of the combination of external and internal cause
and effect. Calluses are a good illustration of this.

Most often caused by the excessive consumption of hard saturated
fats, specifically from cheese, chicken, eggs, and meat, calluses can tell
us what organ is overwhelmed by the accumulation of dense hardened
fats. The skin on the feet thickens and hardens in response to this accumulation, showing the inhibition of organ function in specific organs.

Calluses on the outside of the large toe show an aggravated spleen,
indicating the excessive consumption of sugar and other sweet indulgences. Calluses on the inside of the large toe show that the liver is

kely from the excessive consumption of chicken,
ellfish. If the second and third toes develop calluses,
onding to excessive fat in the diet, while hardened,
the fourth toe shows an aggravated gallbladder. If the
a callus, the bladder and reproductive organs are ac-
ned fat. Finally, a callus that develops on the ball of the
non today, shows that the kidneys are becoming exhausted from overwork.

Along with the elimination of the foods that cause calluses to develop, it's important to have them removed, so that energy can flow freely without blockage through the feet. The removal of calluses from the feet will leave you feeling relaxed and more vital, as energy can be easily absorbed into the body. Once removed, with a diet shift, it will be unlikely that calluses will redevelop. Pedicures are more than just an indulgence to create pretty feet. They can create healthy feet and stronger vitality.

The Toenails

Normally, toenails are a bit harder and thicker than fingernails, as they appear at the lowest peripheral point of the body and, as a result, accumulate more nutrients, which make them tougher.

Normal toenails are slightly darker in color than the fingernails, but like the fingernails, should be smooth and free of ridges or roughness.

If the toenails take on a darker, purplish color, this shows an imbalance in nutrition, caused by extremes in the diet, bouncing from simple sugars to meat and eggs. This condition shows that circulation is inhibited due to mineral-deficient blood from sugar or caused by constricted arteries and veins from a buildup of saturated fats.

If the toenails grow rugged with ridges or thick and white, the liver, gallbladder, and kidneys are overwhelmed with the job of trying to discharge dairy products, fats, and oils in our diet.

The Soles of the Feet

We consider them just the bottoms of our feet. We stand on them all day, run around on them, and massage them when they're tired. Consider this . . . when we stand for long periods on our feet, it's as though our whole body gets tired. Well, it does. The soles of our feet correspond to our entire body, reflecting the health and function of all our major organs.

When the soles of the feet are supple and smooth, free of calluses, dry skin, or other abnormalities, we feel great. These are the feet of someone whose organs are efficiently and smoothly working and whose health and vitality are generally sound.

When specific areas of the sole show hardening, stiffness, or are painful when pressure is applied, it shows that the corresponding organs or systems are in disorder. Calluses or hardness indicate that the organs' functions are sluggish, while pain shows that the organs are aggravated and overworked.

Keeping the soles of the feet soft and elastic is achieved by, of course, eating a balanced diet, as well as taking care of our feet. Therapies like massage, reflexology (acupressure on the feet to relieve pain in other parts of the body), and moxibustion (burning of medicinal herbs near the skin to treat various disorders, used in Chinese medicine) can help to restore the organs and systems of our body to normal, efficient function, and health.

A final point on using your feet to look at your health. There are two specific diagnosis points used in massage that can be very telling for us. Look at your feet and find the small valley formed by the junction of the bones extending from the first and second toes. If this point is painful when pressure is applied, the stomach and liver are aggravated, and the cause is overeating and excessive intake of fluids. The second point of diagnosis is the small valley between the junction of the bones extending from the fourth and fifth toes. If pain is the result of pressure here, it shows that the gallbladder and bladder are aggravated due to the excessive consumption of salts and fats. Adjustments in our eating habits will quickly result in pain-free feet.

Makes you want to baby those little puppies of yours, doesn't it?

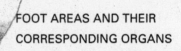

FOOT AREAS AND THEIR
CORRESPONDING ORGANS

a. Spleen   h. Bladder

b. Liver   i. Throat

c. Stomach   j. Abdomen

d. Gallbladder   k. Lower abdomen

e. Bladder   l. Liver, gallbladder (right foot)

f. Spleen   Spleen, pancreas (left foot)

g. Lungs   m. Upper abdomen

Glow-rious Nails

O ur hands are essential tools in communication, and they tell more about us than we know. Our fingernails are an integral part of the hands and a good barometer of our health. We pay a great deal of attention to our nails these days, to the point where they have become, for many, works of art. We want beautiful, strong nails, and we'll do anything to get them, even applying artificial ones to simulate the health that we desire.

Nails are not unlike our hair. They are the result of the discharge of nutrients from the body. With a composition similar to that of our hair, our nails are primarily composed of keratin, the same protein that is the foundation for both skin and hair, although they have a harder, more condensed structure.

Our nails depend on our blood for nutrients, with the quality of our blood affecting their health and appearance. It's no surprise that the quality of the nutrients that feed our nails determines whether they are our pride and joy, or whether we spend a lot of money on nail products, and gloves.

THE STRUCTURE OF NAILS

The hard part of the nail that is most visible is called the nail plate. The tender skin underneath the nail is the nail bed. Our nails grow from the base, known as the matrix, the visible part of which is known as the moon of the nail. While the matrix is where living cells produce the nail bed, the hard nail plate is not composed of living cells. The tender skin that grows around the matrix or base of the nail is the cuticle. The nail bed, the skin under the nail, has blood vessels running through it. These vessels, showing through the translucent nail plate and feeding the production of cells at the matrix, are what ultimately show as the health and appearance of the nail.

Our nails' appearance is influenced by what we choose to eat and drink. The quality of our choices determines the quality of blood that nourishes our organ functions, which in turn are reflected in our nails. Our nails, then, reflect our overall vitality.

Constitution of the Nails

Like the rest of our bodies, our nails possess their inherent character, the traits we are born with, and like the rest of our bodies, the nails show the condition that we create with our daily choices. The constitution of our nails is determined largely by what nourished us while we were in the womb and, it is said, reflects our basic character and tendencies.

Square-shaped nails are reflective of a more contracted constitution, created by the consumption of stronger animal products, cooked vegetables, and salt by the mother during pregnancy. It is said that this nail shape reflects a person who is physically active but can tend to be stubborn.

Oblong-shaped nails are reflective of a mother's diet that included cooked grains and vegetables, fresh foods, and fruits, with animal foods and salt playing a smaller role in the diet. It is said that these nails reflect a person who balances physical activity with rest, but who has very definite ideas about how things should be.

Oval-shaped nails are reflective of a mother's diet that had mostly cooked vegetables as the base, fruit and dairy foods as the supplements. It is said that these nails reflect a person that is physically more delicate and emotionally sensitive.

Long nail plates are reflective of a diet that relied mostly on raw foods, both vegetables and fruit, with sugar and other sweets included. It is said that these nails reflect a person who has a delicate, easily upset digestive system and is easily emotionally upset as well.

The Nails We Create

The constitution of our nails is what we are born with. After that, our choices determine the health and appearance of them. The texture, color, and overall condition of our nails reflect our choices and the impact of them on our health.

Colorful Nails

The color of our nails reflects the quality of blood that feeds them through the blood that circulates through the nail bed. Varying colors in the nails show different aspects of our health.

Normal healthy nails will be pinkish in color, with a smooth feel to the nail plate, free of ridges and cracks. Pinkish nails show that blood is circulating freely and that our health is generally sound.

If the nails show a reddish-purple color, it is an indication that our overall vitality is waning, due to the excessive consumption of expansive foods, including simple sugars, fruits, tropical foods, fatty fried foods, artificial chemicals, coffee, hot spices, and stimulants. These nails indicate that circulation is slowing due to a weakening internal condition and a tendency toward fatigue, with a lower resistance to illness developing, as digestion and respiration grow sluggish.

If the nails take on a deep, deep red color, this indicates that excessive minerals, cholesterol, and fatty acids are accumulating in the bloodstream from the intake of large quantities of eggs, meat, poultry, and salt. The appearance of this color in our nails shows that the circulation is growing sluggish, with blockages in the arteries. Dry skin and hair often accompany this nail condition.

Pale, whitish nails are an indication that the quality of the blood nourishing them is weak. Usually a sign of weak circulation and anemia, this condition is generally caused by the excessive consumption of simple sugars, fruit and fruit juices, along with chemical sweeteners, which deplete our blood of vital nutrients. It's important to note, however, that this condition can also be caused by the excessive consumption of saturated fats, which constrict the blood vessels, inhibiting the flow of blood to the nail bed. In this case, the blood flow is blocked, not weak. So it's important to know what we're eating to diagnose the condition reflected in our nails.

If the nails take on a yellow cast, they are suffocating, literally. Usually seen only in smokers or in people who constantly color their nails, in both cases, the nails are not receiving nutrients. In the case of smokers, obviously, the blood is not properly oxygenated, weakening it and compromising the "feeding" of the nails. In the case of nail coloring, the suffocation comes from applying the chemicals to the nail plate, virtually blocking the discharge and intake of nutrients.

Various Nail Conditions

We can see the condition of our health with more than just the color. Our nails will show other signs of our internal environment based on our diet and lifestyle choices.

Harder, thicker nails are the result of the consumption of animal protein and fat, with the thickening more evident in the toenails than the fingernails. Protein sinks in the body and blockages of energy will tend to be lower in the body, with the nails of the toes showing the accumulation of fat in the arteries more quickly than in the fingers.

On the other hand, thin, fragile, soft nails are the result of the excessive consumption of expansive foods, like coffee, alcohol, and simple, refined sugars.

If vertical ridges appear on the nails, it indicates that eating lacks balance, particularly with fat and protein. Generally, when this condition shows, it means that our diet lacks proper fat and protein, with an excessive consumption of carbohydrates and salt, inhibiting the assimilation of minerals from our diet. It can also mean that our diet lacks minerals. In either case, this condition shows that the digestive system, liver, and kidneys are sluggish, with inhibited assimilation of nutrients. With these ridges, we most often will feel fatigued and depleted.

If you see little white dots on the nails, this shows the elimination of sugar from the body. Along with other mineral depletion, sugar leaches zinc from our system, resulting in white spots on our nails. Simple sugars, including white sugar, honey, maple syrup, fruit sugar and syrups, artificial sweeteners, and alcohol consumption will show as these telltale little spots. Here's the interesting part. You can look at the spots and determine when you had your little sugar binge and which organ system was most affected by the indulgence.

Remember that the thumb shows the condition of the lungs and large intestines, with the first finger showing the health and function of the large intestine. The second finger shows the function of our circulatory system, with the third finger showing our overall health. The pinky finger shows the health and function of the heart and small intestine. By simply examining our nails, we can see which organ function has been compromised by our intake of simple sugars.

Normal adult nails grow from matrix to tip in six to nine months, so we can revisit our little binges. Indulge in piña coladas and pastries on your vacation three months ago? A quick look at your nails will most likely reveal little white spots right about in the center of the nail. Continued indulgences will result in spot after spot growing out, meaning that your organs are overworking to discharge the unwanted sugars from your system. Along with these unsightly little spots, we most often experience chronic fatigue and lack of focus as zinc continues to be depleted.

Horizontal dents in the nails are interesting and can mean more than one thing, so before jumping to any conclusions about your health, be sure to reflect on your life over the last few months. Primarily, these dents are the result of a dramatic change in our eating patterns, resulting either from a move to a different climate, which requires different eating patterns, or simply a dramatic diet change. These dents can also be caused by extremely chaotic eating patterns that leave the body exhausted. Like with white spots, you can track the change by where it appears on the nail, since nail growth takes about six to nine months from matrix to tip.

The secondary cause of horizontal dents in the nails is emotional trauma, like a tragedy, a dramatic change in living style or location, or some other kind of emotional stress. In any of these instances, when our life and diet settle in a normal, natural pattern for us, these dents will cease to appear.

If your nails split at the tips, this indicates that the body is in internal chaos, from the excessive consumption of expansive foods, like simple sugar, coffee, alcohol, and artificial chemicals. This condition shows that our dietary practices are affecting the health and function of the reproductive and nervous systems, with fat accumulating around the ovaries, uterus, or testicles, inhibiting normal function, along with the slowing of our nervous reactions. If one hand shows the splitting and the other doesn't, then the corresponding ovary or testicle is the one affected.

Nothing is more annoying than peeling nails. Layers of our nails strip away, leaving them ragged and fragile. Caused by chemicals, additives, drugs, and medications, this condition shows that the body is deprived of minerals and other nutrients, leaving us malnourished. Along with this condition of the nails, we most often see indigestion, fatigue, nervousness, insomnia, and overall weakness.

And then there are hangnails, those painful, little pieces of cuticle that detach from the nail bed, leaving our hands sore and unsightly. Largely caused by the excessive consumption of simple sugars and other sweeteners, hangnails can be easily remedied with a return to a more balanced way of eating.

The moons at the matrix of the nail plate are the subject of myth and mysticism, credited with everything from sexual virility to spiritual enlightenment, depending on the culture. In traditional healing arts, it is said that the moons reflect our metabolism. In childhood, everyone shows larger moons on the nails and as we mature into adults, our lifestyle and dietary choices show in the size of the moons. Physically active, fit people, making wise dietary choices, will show moons on more nails than those of us choosing a more sedentary lifestyle. Abnormally large moons, however, show that our overall condition is weakening due to the excessive consumption of sweets.

Feeding the Nails

How do we keep our nails fit? How do we achieve those rosy, pink, lustrous, supple, strong nails that are free of spots, lines, dents, holes, or abnormal coloring?

It will come as no surprise to you that a natural, balanced diet is the clearest path to strong, healthy nails. Like our skin and hair, the health of our nails depends on the quality of nutrients that feed them. The balance of both expansive and contracted elements in our diet is responsible for the proper formation of our nails. Too much animal fat and protein, for example, will leave us with hard and brittle nails, resulting from blocked arteries, while too little fat and protein will result in weak, fragile nails, lacking nutrition.

It's easy to see that dietary extremes, both expansive and contracted, will leave our nails in less than perfect condition. A natural diet based on whole grains, seasonal vegetables and fruits, with beans and bean products, sea plants, and proper quantities of fat will result in strong, healthy nails. Naturally beautiful, healthy nails keep our hands looking as youthful and vital as we feel.

Hair, Your Crowning Glory

O h, how we love our hair. Oh, how we hate our hair. Good hair days versus bad hair days have become, for many, the barometer that determines what kind of life we live. So much of our personality and self-image are bound up in our hair. Our obsession with its beauty has grown to epic proportions, and we spend billions on products to make it strong, lustrous, and irresistible to the touch.

And yet we struggle. Our hair is damaged, dull, tangled, brittle, split—breaking our very spirit as we apply product after product to achieve the splendid hair of television commercials. And how do we get that shiny, soft, thick, sensual hair, besides, of course backlighting and hours in the chair of a professional stylist? The answer is so simple that it's scary.

As with our skin, perfect hair is our birthright. Hair's natural tendency is not to be dry and dull, the plague of our lives, but to be rich and lustrous. However, like our skin, our hair reflects our internal condition of health. When life in our internal environment is balanced, with organs and systems working smoothly and efficiently, our hair is happy and shiny. During times of imbalance, our hair looks the part.

Before we can work our way back to the healthy, shiny hair that is naturally ours, we must first understand it. Like every other aspect of being human, our hair has a constitution and a condition and we must differ between them before we can take steps to create our very best hair.

What's Hair, Anyway?

Hair is the symbol of our overall vitality, or lack of it. Hair reflects the condition of our digestive and reproductive systems, with healthy hair reflecting the smooth, efficient function of both these systems. Lustrous, strong hair shows that our ability to digest food and our sexual vitality are strong and healthy. Think of the role hair plays in sexual attraction; strong, shiny, rich hair has inspired poetry and begs to have fingers run through it.

Strong, lustrous, healthy hair shows that our overall life force—our vitality—is active and efficient. It illustrates basically sound health. It is the foundation that we build our hair's condition upon. Shiny, strong, and healthy is the basic constitution of the hair, with ancestral and environmental influences determining certain characteristics.

Like most of our other basic characteristics, we are born with certain hair traits that are unchangeable, except with chemical processing. Color, thickness, whether curly or straight, fine or coarse, these characteristics are ours at birth. Our parents' and ancestors' dietary practices, as well as our developmental environment are the determining factors in the type of hair we're born with.

Take hair color—natural color, that is—not out of a bottle. Like skin, hair color is influenced by the amount of melanin produced in the hair shaft. Blond hair is created by life in cooler, darker climates, like Northern Europe and Scandinavia, for example, where the sunlight is weaker and less frequent. Also influenced by the consumption of dairy foods, which inhibits melanin's rise to the surface of the hair shaft, blond hair, fair skin, and light eyes are the constitutional traits of that ancestry. Red hair is created by life in cooler, darker climates, like

Ireland, where, with less sunlight, more animal protein is eaten for warmth, creating more iron in the bloodstream. Dark brown and black hair is created in a sunny, warm, more Southern climate, where cooling vegetables and fruits are the feature, with animal foods playing a smaller role in the diet and the bright sun draws more melanin to the surface of the hair shaft.

The texture of the hair, thick, coarse, or fine, as well as whether hair is curly or straight, is also influenced by our ancestors and their dietary practices. Hair that is straight is the result of more vegetables in the diet, while curly hair, which is caused by a tighter hair follicle, is the result of more contracting animal foods in the diet. Wavy hair is the result of a diet that includes both animal and vegetable foods, and is, of course, the most common hair texture we see today. Thick hair is the result of a diet where veggies play a more prominent role in the diet, with coarse hair being the result of more animal protein. Fine hair is the result of a diet rich in dairy foods and sugar, with less animal and vegetable-quality proteins.

After our early formative years, it is up to us to create the condition of our hair, which is greatly influenced by our diet and lifestyle choices. Dry hair, oily hair, brittle, fragile hair, thinning hair, graying hair, dandruff, split ends, all of these conditions of the hair are created, primarily, by what we choose to eat and drink, with minor influences from the environment.

There are two types of hair, the hair on our heads and the hair on our faces and bodies. Both are influenced by differing factors and show differing facets of our health. Expansive influences govern the health and vitality of our head hair, which expands and grows from the top of our head, while more contractive influences govern the health and vitality of face and body hair.

Hair is the result of the nutrients in our diet. Primarily produced from protein, hair production is also influenced by fats, minerals, and carbohydrates. In short, our daily food is transformed into our hair. The growth of hair alternates between active and rest periods, with about 85 percent of the hair actively growing, with about 15 percent at rest, with the ratio between growth and rest being about seven to one, growing being seven times longer than rest. A balanced human diet reflects this same kind of ratio, with a normal diet having a similar ratio of nutrients, with protein ingestion being seven times that of minerals and carbohydrates being seven times more than protein for balance. This balance of nutrients creates the cycles of hair growth. Trying to grow out a short haircut more quickly? Try balancing your diet with these ratios and see the difference. Most women that eat a plant-based diet, balanced within these ratios, complain that their hair grows like weeds.

Our hair also grows in accordance with the seasons. Responding to diet and environmental changes, hair grows and rests as the seasons fluctuate. During summer weather, we tend to eat foods with more expansive natures, vegetables, fruits, and the like. Because of the activity of summer, with intense heat and nature at its most active, we tend to eat less, to make balance with the intensity. Hair is stimulated to active growth as a result of the expansive nature of the season and also to release some of the heat that is being held in the body, also to balance the intensity of the season. So like plants, our hair grows thick and lush in summer weather.

On the other hand, autumn and winter are times of the year when activity is curtailed and the body tries to hold on to its internal warmth. As the weather cools, our energy turns inward and we use all of our resources to hold on to the heat that will balance us with the external cold around us. As our bodies reserve energy, hair growth slows, as the body contracts to conserve energy.

Hair is interesting in how similar it is to plants in structure. As the very life of plants depends on the nutrients absorbed by the soil, our hair relies on the nutrients from our bloodstream for its life and health. Even the structure of the hair shaft is similar to that of plants. There's the shaft, appearing above the skin, the root, just below the surface of the skin, and the bulb that holds the root in place. Each hair has three layers—the cuticle, the outermost layer that suffers the most superficial damage, the cortex, the elastic layer that holds the pigment that colors the hair; and the medulla, the part of the hair that draws nutrients into it. It's not a long stretch to understand then, that our food choices are the most important influence over the quality and health of our hair.

You may be wondering what reproductive function has to do with the health of our hair. In a word, hormones. When reproductive function is balanced and smooth, with our cycles flowing and ebbing with the weeks of the month, we don't see our menstrual cycle as the plague of our lives and our hormones gently fluctuate with our changes. When our diet adversely influences our hormone balance, we experience radical changes in our hair, from oily to dull and dry, depending on what our raging hormones are up to on that particular day.

DIMMING YOUR HAIR'S GLOW

How do we keep hair's natural radiance and health, or regain it once it has been compromised? The bad news is that growing radiant hair is a slow process. Unlike our skin, hair will not immediately reflect positive changes in our diet and lifestyle. Once hair is damaged or destroyed, we must wait for new growth to see the difference.

If we were to look at hair under a microscope, we would see that it has a spiral structure, reflecting all of nature and its own spiral of life, from our fingertips to water sluicing down the drain to hurricane movement to the structure of the DNA that composes life. Reflecting this natural spiral is the structure of our hair. Keratin is the protein that is the main component of the hair shaft, with its molecules forming a seven-strand spiral pattern around a central axis that forms the shaft. Healthy hair is the result of these strands being well formed, complete, without breakage. Well-formed keratin strands are the result of a balanced eating pattern and simple care of the hair.

Like the rest of our body and its functions, our hair craves balance and performs best when the nutrients feeding it are balanced. Extreme foods will leave the hair looking less than healthy for a variety of reasons. Of course, we know that applying chemical solutions to the hair, color, permanent waves, or curl relaxers will damage the protein molecules that wrap around the shaft, leaving hair brittle and dull, but food creates the condition of our hair on a deeper level.

Foods of an extremely expansive nature, like refined sugar, chemicals, strong spices, alcohol, caffeine, and tropical fruit can cause the keratin molecules to break apart, preventing the tight spiraling around the axis that we need for healthy, shiny hair. With excessive consumption of these foods, we find that our hair grows brittle and delicate, easily damaged and broken. On the other hand, excessive consumption of animal proteins and fats, salt, and other constricting foods will leave the hair damaged from malnutrition, as the blood capillaries constrict, preventing the flow of blood and nutrients to the hair shaft, leaving hair looking lifeless, starved for nourishment.

That's the external part of the hair, but there's more to it. Our hair is reflective of our health in a very specific way and balancing the function of our digestive and reproductive systems will ensure strong, lustrous hair, and the end of bad hair days. When we choose foods that tax the delicate balance that our digestive tract craves, we create any number of internal plagues that result in less than beautiful hair.

Dry Hair

Is there anything worse than dry hair, that brittle, fragile, dull nest on our heads that requires gobs of moisturizing products to simulate the appearance of the glossy tresses that we crave?

Dry hair is the result of excessive consumption of saturated fats that harden in the body, veins, and arteries. This is a gradual process, building over years of consumption of animal fats and proteins; we don't wake up one day with dry hair. We see it build up over time, often attributing our dry hair to our aging process. In fact, dry hair happens when the body can no longer discharge our excesses efficiently and the fats and proteins we continue to eat begin to gather and accumulate. With our dry hair, we may also see that our skin is growing harder and drier. What is actually happening is that our glands and oil ducts have become completely clogged and are unable to receive moisture, leaving our skin and hair dehydrated, dry, and malnourished.

Of course, the excessive consumption of salt or the use of processed salts, processed foods, and the insufficient intake of vegetable oils and fluids can contribute to dry hair, as can the use of chemical solutions for color, waving, and relaxing curl, but the primary cause of dry hair is the buildup of saturated fat in our bodies that effectively block nutrients and moisture reaching the hair shaft.

Oily Hair

Oily hair can often be caused by the excessive consumption of saturated fats, but in that case, oily hair is the precursor to dry hair, with the oil of the saturated fats being discharged through the hair shaft, leaving the ends of the hair dry and brittle and the roots oily.

However, many people who don't eat a lot of animal foods suffer from oily hair. Oily hair is very often caused by the excessive intake of vegetable oils, fried foods, chips, and other sources of oil, like nuts and nut butters, in our diet. On the other end of the spectrum, the excessive use of simple or refined sugars will also contribute to oily hair. Turning quickly to fat in the body, simple sugars, like white sugar, honey, fruits, and fruit juices will be actively discharged through the skin and hair, resulting in oily, limp hair. Whether animal foods, simple sugar, or dense vegetable fats, oily hair is the result of the buildup of fat in the body, under the skin and in the vessels and arteries.

Ironically, with oily hair, we take the exact action that makes the condition worse. Rather than a dietary adjustment that, over time, will reduce the production of oil that creates this condition, we shampoo and shampoo and shampoo. This kind of excessive cleansing will actually stimulate the production of oil that the hair shaft needs to remain soft and shiny. The result is hair that dries and splits at the ends and continues to grow oily at the roots. A diet change, along with more gentle cleansing, will yield the internal balance that will create shiny, sensual hair.

Split Ends

When the keratin strands that wrap around the axis of the hair shaft break apart, splitting and fraying occur at the ends of the hair. Split ends are basically the breakdown of the hair shaft. The primary cause of split ends is the excessive consumption of expansive foods, like fruit, sugars, raw foods, and salads. These kinds of extremes in the diet cause the ends of the hair to fray in several ways. The very nature of expansive foods, when eaten in excess, will prevent the keratin from contracting and wrapping around the hair shaft effectively, resulting in the splitting of the strands. In addition, extremes of expansive foods will leach minerals and other nutrients from the hair, leaving it starved and weak, finally fraying as it continues to degenerate.

Consuming large quantities of simple, refined sugars, including honey, maple syrup and chemical sweeteners, soft drinks, strong spices, ice cream, frozen yogurt, drugs, and other chemicals contribute to both causes of split ends, as they weaken the molecular bonding of the hair.

While saturated fats can contribute to the condition by inhibiting the flow of nutrients to the entire hair shaft, as can the application of chemical solutions to the surface of the shaft, they are, by far, minor causes. The overwhelming cause of split ends is sugars and chemical additives that weaken and starve the hair from root to tip.

Dandruff

Peeling and flaking of the scalp, dandruff, is a problem of epidemic proportions. Product after product promise "no more flakes," but still we struggle with this condition.

Normally, skin cells are sloughed off the surface of the skin as they come to the surface, in a natural exfoliation, revealing fresh skin to the world. In normal skin conditions, these cells have such a fine powder-like texture that they are virtually undetected. In the case of dandruff, however, these tiny, fine cells clump together, forming coarse, white scales. Over time, if left unchecked, dandruff will worsen, with the scalp growing red and irritated and spreading to other parts of the body, like the sides of the nose, eyebrows, eyelids, near the navel, groin, and possibly the upper back.

Although we think of dandruff as dry flakes, dandruff is actually oil and protein clumping together. And our typical, topical solution? We apply creamy products to our scalp to solve the problem, but these applications only "glue" the flakes to the scalp, delaying their falling away, actually aggravating the problem by creating more blockage on the surface of the skin.

Dandruff is essentially the elimination of excess fat and protein building up in the body. Although overeating can contribute to the condition, dandruff is essentially caused by the excessive consumption of the saturated fats and proteins in animal foods, with fried foods as a contributing cause. As with other conditions of the hair, dandruff is caused by oil and protein clogging the glands and follicles, eventually clumping together, blocking discharge and intake of moisture to the skin of the scalp. The result is that the skin cells, which would normally slough off the surface of the skin, clump together, bound by oil, and form the large flakes we recognize as dandruff.

Hair on the Face and Body

Hair on the face and body mean different things to different people, particularly men and women. The hair on the face and body indicate opposite conditions in men and in women.

Before going any further, however, it is important to note that facial and body hair vary in many cultures. For instance, Native Americans, Asians, and people of African heritage, as well as some Northern European people, do not grow thick body and facial hair. This will prove meaningful as we examine the causes of irregularities in hair growth on the face and body.

Facial and body hair is produced when the male hormone, androgen, is stimulated to production. In men, this hormone is responsible for moustaches, beards, chest, and other body hair. Again, while this may vary culturally, strong facial and body hair, or facial and body hair that is uniform in growth, is an indication that they are sexually vital and strong, with efficient reproductive function.

Androgen is also present in women and the stimulation of its production, in excess, will produce the same characteristics we admire in our men, moustaches, excess body hair, and in some cases, even a light beard.

In both men and women, facial and body hair is produced by the discharge of strong protein, in particular, eggs, hard cheese, shellfish, and red meat. Excessive consumption of these foods will cause the excessive production of facial and body hair, in women, in particular. The intake of strongly contracting foods, like animal proteins and fats, stimulate the adrenal glands to produce androgen, in the case of women, more than we need. This hormone production results in the growth of facial and excessive amounts of body hair.

The upper lip, the area of the face between the nose and top lip, reflects the health and function of the reproductive system. In men, when we see strong, uniform facial hair here, we know that this man is producing strong male hormones, resulting in vitality in the reproductive system. In women, on the other hand, hair growth on the upper lip means that she is consuming excessive amounts of protein, creating hormonal imbalance, caused by the excessive production of androgen. It also indicates that excessive fat and protein are accumulating around the ovaries and uterus. It is a condition that demands our attention, as our reproductive health is at stake.

Excessive body hair in women is also an indication that excessive amounts of protein are being consumed, causing the protein to discharge from various organs and systems as body hair.

In many women, we also see the growth of a fine, down-like hair that grows on the cheeks and along the jawline. Caused by the excessive consumption of dairy foods, these silvery hairs indicate that the kidneys and lungs are clogged with accumulated congestion and are growing weak. Along with this fine down, we usually see a very pale, almost white complexion. In Chinese medicine, it's said that this fine hair represents the body's attempt to protect its weakening organs.

One final word on body hair concerns that found on the back. Rarely seen in women, back hair has a very specific meaning in men, especially when a man is carpeted on his back with hair. While strong facial and chest hair mean that the secretion of androgen is strong in men, hair on the back is actually indicative of a growing weakness. As with the fine down we sometimes find on women's faces, hair on the shoulders and back indicate that the lungs (in the instance of shoulder blade and upper back hair) and the intestines (with shoulder hair) are growing weak and the body is trying to protect these weakening organs with outside insulation, just like animals' coats thickening with cold weather. In the case of excess body hair in these areas, you most often also find that the person stands with stooped shoulders, a protective stance, seemingly trying to shield the weakened lungs from the onslaught of life.

Losing Our Hair

Hair loss has become an epidemic in humanity, even in women. We see product after product, both prescription and over-the-counter, promising to grow the hair we are rapidly losing.

Baldness is a condition that is easily avoided in life. Normally, we lose somewhere between fifty and a hundred hairs daily, which are replaced by new growth. When the loss exceeds the regrowth, we see baldness. Diet and lifestyle (as well as genetics) play important roles in whether or not you will hold on to your hair, and it has little to do with family history. The common link between families and baldness is shared eating patterns that are passed from generation to generation, as are our preferences and predispositions to conditions. A diet and lifestyle change can break the pattern of generations of baldness.

Baldness has three basic causes and will occur in certain patterns. Hair loss that begins at the front of the head is the result of too many expansive influences in the diet, with the hairline receding until most of the frontal hair is gone or substantially thinned. The excessive consumption of foods with an expansive nature causes the hair follicles to open and the hair is lost. It literally cannot stay rooted in the scalp, since the follicle is so expanded. Caused by the excessive intake of fluids, including tropical fruit juices, soft drinks, diet soda, simple sugars, chemical sweeteners, chemical additives, drugs and medication, and excessive use of raw tomatoes, potatoes, and eggplant, these foods cause the blood to become overly acidic, weakening the kidneys and liver, inhibiting the hair follicles' ability to contract and hold the hair in place. Along with this type of baldness, it is not uncommon to see diabetes, hypoglycemia, and anemia as accompanying chronic conditions.

The second pattern of baldness occurs at the center of the head, at the top, and is caused by the excessive consumption of contracting or constricting foods. Consuming large quantities of animal protein and fat causes two things to happen that can ultimately result in baldness. Contracting foods do exactly that, contract. These kinds of foods also "sink" in the body, creating deep strength but also inhibiting energy from rising in the body. For hair to grow on the head, our life energy must rise, along with nutrients to "feed" the growth.

Along with drawing nutrients from the scalp, animal proteins and fats also cause the follicles on the scalp to shut down, as the follicles clog with saturated fat, literally choking off the hair, so it drops out. At the same time, animal proteins stimulate the production of male hormones, which in turn stimulate the production of facial and body hair, while the overwork involved in the digestion of these foods weaken and exhaust our internal organs, hence the balding head and hairy back.

In women, interestingly, it is the increase in animal foods in our diet that has caused the rise of thinning hair in us, as well as in men. The production of testosterone and androgen are stimulated by the excessive consumption of eggs, cheese, red meat, poultry, even shellfish. In turn, these hormones stimulate the production of facial and body hair, while stifling the production of head hair. As women consume more and more animal foods, we will be plagued by baldness at the same alarming rate as men.

The final pattern of baldness is caused by a combination of extreme foods from both ends of the spectrum. This is the baldness that occurs over a large region of the head, covering the sides, top, and front areas of the head, leaving a ring of hair around the head, with perhaps a few strands lingering at the top.

Caused by the excessive consumption of both simple sugars and chemicals and animal fats and proteins, as well as a lack of minerals, this pattern of baldness is the result of both the loosening of the follicles that drop hair and the choking off of the follicles, also dropping hair. As the extremes of that kind of eating pattern take their toll on our internal organs, working them to exhaustion, baldness is just one of the results.

Baldness doesn't have to become yet another plague to struggle with in life. A balanced diet can remove the shadow of this condition. That's the good news. Theory tells us that anything is possible, and I have had people tell me that they have seen the growth of new hair with dietary changes. More important than your appearance, however, if you find that your hair is thinning, your internal environment needs your attention; you can worry about your appearance after your health is back on track.

Gray Hair

We fight gray hair with every ounce of strength. We pluck them, color them, do anything to hide them. And while they're inevitable, for many of us they show up long before they should.

Hair color comes from melanocytes, cells of the hair shaft that conduct color to our hair. The branchlike structures, dendrites, which are attached to these cells secrete the pigment that is absorbed into newly formed hair cells, that shows as the color in our hair. Gray hair is the result of these cells growing dry, constricted, and shriveled, which occurs when the blood vessels that feed the hair grow constricted, inhibiting the flow of nutrients to the hair shaft. Inhibiting the secretion of pigment results in less color, or no color, gray or white hair.

Caused primarily by the consumption of saturated fat and protein, as well as salt, coupled with a lack of vegetables in the diet, gray hair is a sign that our hair is starving. A secondary cause of graying hair is the excessive intake of simple sugars, which leach minerals from the blood, weakening the nutrients that reach the hair, and the melanocytes' ability to secrete color is compromised. The more foods we consume that are either lacking in nutrients and life, or depleting to our systems, the sooner we'll see gray hair in our lives. Premature gray hair, that is graying before we reach late middle age, is a sign that our food is not properly nourishing us. We're starving, malnourished from the excessive intake of foods that overwork and deplete us. Along with premature gray hair, we most often see that these people are chronically tired, lacking in energy.

Gray hair is, however, natural as we age. Part of the aging process is that we don't assimilate minerals as well as we do in our youth. As we lose or don't assimilate minerals, again, the melanocytes weaken in their ability to secrete pigment to the hair shaft, resulting in gray hair. Gray hair is normal at this phase of life, not necessarily a sign of malnutrition. As we age, we require less food, less sleep, move a bit more slowly, and live more in rhythm with our natural cycles. With a healthy approach to eating and moderate exercise, our later lives can be as vital and strong as our youth. At this point, those white hairs are a sign of maturity, wisdom, and experience. Perhaps we shouldn't be so quick to turn them over to color in a bottle.

HEALTHY, GLOWING HAIR

The health of our hair relies heavily on the health of our digestive tract. Closely related to the health of the microvilli in the intestine as well as the digestive system as a whole, our hair's health depends on how well food is digested and nutrients absorbed.

It should come as no surprise that the fiber in whole grains is essential to the health of our digestive tract, and our hair. Promoting the smooth elimination of waste, fiber prevents accumulation in the intestines that can result in the formation of toxins. On top of that, soluble fiber, like that found in whole grains, can help to lower cholesterol, which impacts on the health of the hair directly. When cholesterol levels in the blood are normal, our blood circulates freely, with no blockages, feeding the hair efficiently and thoroughly. Finally, being complex carbohydrates, whole grains feed the blood with nutrients, unlike simple carbohydrates that leach minerals and vitamins from the bloodstream, leaving us feeling depleted and our hair dull and tired.

Fermented foods and pickles are also ideal hair food. Among these foods are soy sauce, tamari, and miso, with miso being the most beneficial to our hair. Made from soybeans, whole grain, and salt, miso is fermented over a period of several months or years, and is rich in living enzymes that ease digestion, fortify the quality of the blood nourishing the body and hair, and provide us with essential oils, vitamins, and minerals.

Pickled foods have been used throughout history to stimulate the appetite, improve digestion, and strengthen the digestive tract. Pickled vegetables, including natural sauerkraut, aid the intestines in the process of feeding our hair.

Most important for maintenance of our hair's health is the consumption of small quantities of sea plants. Eaten on a daily basis, these simple plants are rich in the nutrients most essential for maintaining healthy, shiny hair, free of split ends. Used by many cultures as food, sea plants are also essential ingredients in many natural shampoos and can be used to fortify damaged hair, until new growth shows the changes in our diet.

Rich in beta-carotene, sea plants help to prevent the buildup of dead skin cells that can clog the hair follicles, inhibiting the growth and health of the hair. The B vitamins, also found in sea plants, have been linked to the prevention of oily hair, baldness, and dandruff. Also rich in calcium (essential to the structure of the hair shaft), phosphorous, potassium, sulphur, magnesium, copper (which aids in giving color to the hair), selenium, bromine, and others, sea plants are a key food for preventing premature gray hair.

It only gets better with sea plants. Seawater, in combination with sea plants, neutralizes toxins in the sea. Eating sea plants will have the same effect on our bloodstream, with the minerals in the plants working to harmonize our internal imbalances. Aiding the body in elimination of excessive sugars, saturated fats, and other acid-producing foods, sea plants efficiently cleanse the blood, so that the nutrients that get to the hair shaft are pure and strong.

The combination of firmness, flexibility, strength from growing in seawater, along with being rich resources of nutrients make sea plants the ideal hair food, helping to prevent many of the woes we struggle with, as well as contributing to the strong, lustrous hair we think we can find only on television.

30-Day Plan to
Glowing Radiance

Everybody loves a plan. While every bone in my body screams to release you from "plans," so that you are able to take back responsibility for your own health with freedom, I have come to realize that, as we have grown more detached from nature, we have grown more detached from our intuitive knowledge about making peace with our environment. Living in harmony with our surroundings has become nothing more than a cliché that we bandy about without understanding what it means, or how good it feels to actually live that way.

We live in a time when every self-proclaimed expert under the sun wants to tell you what's best for you. And as more and more experts are paraded in front of us, each heralding his or her plan as "the answer," we grow more confused. There's a reason for that. There is only one expert in your life: you. There is only one person who knows exactly what it is that you need to live in harmony with your world: you. The advice offered by experts can be sound and thoughtful, but the wise person will filter the information through the brain and apply to his or her life that which is appropriate.

My 30-Day Plan to Glowing Radiance is a plan without a plan. Think of it as a set of guidelines with the purpose of showing you simple ways to create harmony in your life, divided into three categories: diet, lifestyle, and self-care. Which one is most important? Only you can decide.

While not big on guarantees, I will say that if you follow these simple guidelines and imprint them in appropriate ways onto your own unique life, you will find yourself glowing, your natural radiance and vitality freed from the constraints of imbalance, revealing the dazzling, inherent beauty that is your birthright. Try it, for thirty days. You and the world will be better for it.

DIET TO GLOW BY

It's probably obvious that I believe that the quality of foods we choose on a daily basis influence the health and vitality of our bodies. While it may not be the sole determinant of whether or not we are healthy, it is one of the most important, and it is the one over which we exercise control. We decide what we eat.

In the fifth century, B.C., Hippocrates, the philosopher said to be the father of Western medicine, coined the famous oath, ". . . let food be thy medicine and let medicine be thy food . . ." While not exactly in fashion in our modern culture, food and healing were very much entwined in more ancient times but have been relegated to the world of folklore today. From chicken soup for a cold, to garlic for lung congestion and purifying the blood, to ginger for circulation and the discharge of toxins and stomach upset and pickles for digestion, food and its energy have always been revered and used for their ability to balance and normalize our health. An understanding of the power of food in our life enables us to utilize food in all its delicious glory to create the life and health we want.

Not a fan of deprivation, I think that it's essential that your change in thinking about food is viewed as positive, an adventure in new culinary experiences, rather than a grim litany chanted in your head daily of what you are no longer eating. While I'm not espousing a life of tofu and bean sprouts, I will firmly state that the only thing to be gained by a diet rich in saturated fats and animal protein is weight and heart disease (among other things).

Whole, natural foods that are well prepared are both delicious and satisfying to the body and soul. I come from an Italian heritage and richness runs in my blood. No matter what, I can't subsist on a diet of steamed vegetables, boiled foods, and no fat. And to avoid dessert would be like avoiding life itself. What I have discovered in my own culinary adventures is that I have come full circle in my approach to healthy cooking. When I drastically changed my diet to cope with my health crisis, I went from a diet rich in simple sugars and fats to a diet that could only be described as austere. My health recovered, I went on to rebel (a natural state of being for me), and started searching for ways to make cooking seem rich again. From there, my evolution has currently taken me back to my ancestral roots, where I have made my peace. I have learned to fuse the understanding I've gained about food and its energy, with my heritage and have discovered that they differ very little after all.

My Italian mother taught me two important principles in cooking that ensure success in meal preparation as well as health. She said that the importance of ingredients, what she called "materia prima," was essential to creating a delicious meal that would satisfy the body on all levels. With poor quality ingredients, she would lecture, you must complicate the dishes, to disguise the inferior nature of the food. How apt is her advice in my current approach to cooking!

The second principle not to be ignored, she told me, as she gently stirred and sautéed, was simple presentation. She believed that showing food in its naturally beautiful state was all that was necessary to create appeal. Again, she was right. She never chose canned vegetables or processed foods for her meals. As a child, I never understood her obsession with freshness. It was more than inconvenient to travel with her from market to market in search of the freshest ingredients. I was aware, however, of how delicious her food was to me. It wasn't until my own evolution that I connected the dots. I'm so grateful to her for instilling that standard of excellence in me. I often wonder if she knew how well I would use her words of advice.

Food that is of excellent quality and in its whole, natural state requires very little adornment to appeal to us. Simple foods that are well prepared have an elegance that cannot be improved upon. So your food choices, as well as making the choice to prepare the foods you'll be eating, are essential to your health and radiance.

If cooking and visual appeal aren't enough incentive for you to make a change in your food choices, there are other, perhaps more tangible ones. Just a short while after making more appropriate food choices, you'll find that you feel stronger, more vital and have more stamina. You'll sleep more soundly and wake refreshed. You'll think more clearly and find that you handle life's daily crises more calmly. You'll find that you have less aches and pains, more flexibility in your muscles and joints, better digestion, and a more positive attitude. Your skin and hair condition will improve, your eyes will be clearer, and you won't tire as easily. You'll look and feel like a new person.

More than all of the physical improvements that come with healthy food choices, we discover what creates the energy that flows through us, enlivening both nature and us. That understanding of the energy of life is worth the price of admission.

FOODS THAT DIM YOUR GLOW

While we've talked about the foods that rob us of vitality, it's important to see them all together, as guidelines. Remember that there are no "good" or "bad" foods, only foods that serve us and those that don't.

1. Avoid red meat. Red meats are high in saturated fats and cholesterol and are not really necessary to our existence. With more than half their calories coming from fat, red meats are an inefficient fuel that consumes tremendous amounts of our resources to digest them. Compromising digestion, clogging arteries, and contributing to dry skin and hair, animal proteins and fats are not high on the list of foods to glow by.

2. Avoid dairy products. High in saturated fat and protein, dairy products are about as unnatural a food choice as we can make. Nature created milk for each species to nourish and support the life of its young. Chemically and energetically, these foods are designed by nature to meet those needs, to grow the young of each species. There are two conclusions to draw here: one, that to drink milk from another species is not natural, and second, that to cross species and drink the milk of another creates biological

turmoil. However, if that's a bit too esoteric for your taste, try this: The protein available to us in milk is extremely dense and utilizes a great deal of resources to assimilate it. Add to that weight gain and pasty skin and, look at it this way, when we stop nursing, we should stop nursing.

3. Avoid eggs. With one egg containing 250 milligrams of cholesterol and 64 percent of its calories from fat, eggs can be tough on our bodies. Hard to digest, but helpful in the weight gain department, eggs make us feel bulky and create stiff muscles and joints. Eggs are a great source of vitamin B-12, but I think that there are better ways to get this vitamin, but there you are.

4. Avoid poultry. Not much better for us than red meats, poultry, especially chicken, is an extreme food and best to be avoided if we want to look our best. Poultry meat is one of the densest forms of protein, second only to eggs, and is difficult to digest. Poultry has a layer of thick fat just under the skin, just like the layer of fat it causes under our own, resulting in dry skin, blemishes, and dandruff. They don't call loose, aging flesh "chicken skin" for nothing.

5. Avoid refined sugars and flour. These foods serve absolutely no purpose and have no regular place in our diet. Hard to avoid when eating in restaurants, these foods leach minerals from our bloodstream, clog the intestines, causing them to swell and grow weak, cause weight gain and lethargy, and cloud our thinking.

Being a realist, I know that most people aren't going to clean out their cupboards and dive headlong into healthy eating. I recommend, however, that you reduce your intake of foods that don't support your life and see how you feel. The better you feel, the more you'll try.

FOODS FOR GLOWING RADIANCE

What do we eat to ensure that our vitality is strong and we put our best face forward every day? I think it's important to say, again, that eating well doesn't mean eating a grim regime of steamed vegetables. Whole, fresh foods that are well prepared are as delicious as any fussy dish you can imagine. It may take a few weeks to re-enliven your taste buds to the subtleties in tastes of foods in their natural state, but it's worth it. Once your mouth has come alive again, the flavors of the most simple of ingredients literally bursts on your tongue.

A truly healthy diet is wide and varied, featuring a selection of grains, beans, seasonal vegetables and fruits, pickled foods, condiments, superior-quality fats and sweets, and for those who choose it, fish. The proportions of any variety of foods you eat needs to be based on your own health condition, your goals, and your dreams for your life.

Whole Grains

The centerpiece of a whole-foods diet, whole grains are power-houses of energy. Whole grains are grains that have not been stripped of their fiber, germ, and bran, retaining the majority of their nutrients.

Before you panic, thinking that this is the part where I doom you to a life of brown rice and seaweed, relax. I would never do that to you. Without variety, there is no way we can maintain interest in any eating pattern; it's the key to enjoyment, and the key to health. Nature has provided us with so many sources of nutrients that to limit our food choices to only a few items would be foolish.

Amaranth	**Oats**	Red
	Rolled	Short, medium, and
Barley	Steel-cut	long-grain
	Whole	Sweet
Buckwheat (kasha)		Wehani
	Quinoa	**Teff**
Corn		
	Rice	**Wheat**
Millet	Arborio	Bulgur
	Basmati	Couscous
	Mochi (a sweet brown	Whole-wheat berries
	rice cake)	

Along with all of these, and other grains and grain products, we also choose from whole-grain and semolina pasta, whole-grain breads, flat breads, tortillas, and chapatis.

Beans and Bean Products

Beans provide us with protein, complex carbohydrates, and other essential nutrients. More important, they provide us with a slow-burning energy, like putting our burner on simmer, so that we have reserves of vitality to draw on to keep ourselves going through the day with even levels of stamina.

Adzuki	**Green**	**Tofu**
	Le Puy	Fresh
Black turtle	Red	Dried
Black-eyed peas		Frozen
	Lima	**Tempeh**
Fava (broad)		
	Pinto	
Kidney		**Split peas**
		Green
Lentils	**Soybeans**	Yellow
Brown	Black	
Black	Yellow	

In addition to these choices for beans, there are numerous others that I haven't mentioned, so choose what suits your taste, culture, and desire. And for those who choose it, fish is an excellent source of protein, omega-3 oils, B vitamins, and other vital nutrients. Just take care in choosing wild or fresh fish rather than farm-raised fish, which can contain contaminants and antibiotics.

Vegetables

Nature has provided us with such an array of abundance that I am in awe. Each time I stand in a market with bins overflowing with the season's harvest I'm inspired with a renewed passion for cooking. There is so much for us to choose from, I sometimes feel like there aren't enough meals to prepare them all.

Green vegetables	Carrot greens	Dandelion
Asparagus	Chinese cabbage	Endive
Bok choy	Collard greens	Belgian
Broccoli rabe	Daikon greens	Curly

Escarole

Frisée

Kale

Kohlrabi

Leeks

Lettuce

Mustard greens

Parsley

Scallions

Shepherd's purse

Sorrel

Sprouts

Turnip greens

Watercress

Ground vegetables

Artichokes

Broccoli

Brussels sprouts

Cabbage

Green

Red

Cauliflower

Celery

Cucumber

Fennel

Green beans

Green peas

Mushrooms

Okra

Squash

Acorn

Buttercup

Butternut

Delicata

Hokkaido pumpkin

Hubbard

Red kuri

Pumpkin

Snow peas

Sweet potatoes

Yams

Yellow summer squash

Zucchini

Root Vegetables

Burdock

Carrots

Chicory root

Daikon radish

Lotus root

Parsnips

Red radishes

Rutabaga

Salsify root

Turnips

As for the nightshade vegetables, tomato, potato, green pepper, and eggplant, using them in small amounts is wisest. I would also advise that they always be cooked, dried, marinated, stewed, or roasted, prepared in some way to neutralize their acidic nature. It's that acid that aggravates arthritic conditions, weakens the blood, and leaves us feeling less than our best. And while I'm a firm believer in the theory that no vegetable will kill us, and while I use these strong vegetables on occasion for their extreme qualities, I also believe that vegetables as strongly acidic as these serve us best when cooked well and used less frequently than the list of other vegetables shown here.

Sea Plants

I know, here it comes, the dreaded sea plants. Actually considered to be somewhat exotic these days, sea plants are coming into the mainstream. Their dramatic colors, strong, distinct flavors, and interesting textures lend themselves to a variety of preparations. The most important factor in choosing sea vegetables, however, is their nutritional value to us and to our radiant glow.

Agar

Arame

Dulse

Hiziki

Kombu/Kelp

Nori

Sea palm

Wakame/Alaria

A mere five percent of the diet, taken as sea plants, will provide us with many of the essential vitamins and minerals we need to feel and look our best.

Soups

While not a food group, soup is one of the most important eating choices you can make. Served as the first course of a meal, soup relaxes the digestive tract, so that we can digest our food more efficiently and easily. Eaten every day, at one or two meals, soup can help you feel centered, relaxed, and satisfied.

Fruits and Desserts

As I say in the dessert chapter, desserts and sweet flavors are an important part of a healthy diet. Including them in our daily repertoire of foods helps us to relax, prevents us from overeating and binging, and helps us to feel satisfied with our eating patterns. A small, good-quality treat will go a long way toward keeping us on an even keel. Wouldn't it be nice to be free of the slavery to sugar?

FRUIT (CHOOSE SEASONALLY)

Apples	Figs	Plums
Apricots	Grapes	Raspberries
Blackberries	Lemons	Strawberries
Blueberries	Limes	Tangerines
Cantaloupe	Pears	Dried fruits

Of course, these are choices for a temperate climate. For those of us living in tropical climates, we can choose from oranges, mangoes, papayas, bananas, grapefruit, and all the other luscious fruits that are abundant in these climes. In temperate zones, we want to keep these fruits to a minimum, as they can cool our bodies more than we want to be cooled in the erratic weather of the four seasons.

DESSERTS (MADE WITH GRAIN, NUT AND SOY MILKS, AND WHOLE-GRAIN FLOURS AND SWEETENERS)

Amasake

Cakes

Cookies

Custards

Pies

Puddings

When made with superior ingredients, desserts can feed us body and soul.

Seasonings

Seasonings can make or break any meal. Choosing from a variety of condiments brings balance to a meal, adds sparkle to a simple dish, and brings out the naturally delicious character of your ingredients.

A sprinkle, a dash, a pinch, all the little details we know as seasoning, are the keys to creating meals that dance on your tongue and leave you feeling satisfied and content.

Barley or brown rice miso	**Ginger**	**Sesame oil**
(naturally aged for		**Light**
	Horseradish	
18 months)		**Toasted**
	Mirin	
Brown rice vinegar		**Soy sauce (naturally aged**
	Olive oil	**for a minimum of**
Chile peppers		**18 months)**
	Sea salt	
Fresh and dried herbs	**(unrefined)**	**Umeboshi plums**
Garlic		**Umeboshi plum vinegar**

Nuts and Seeds

Nuts and seeds provide us with a tremendous number of nutrients. Delicious, rich, and satisfying, nuts are a great source of energy and vitality, as well as being an excellent source of fat in our lean diet. Their crunch adds variety to our eating, their flavor is heavenly, and their energy is priceless.

A handful here, a sprinkle over grain, that unexpected bit of crunch in a cookie, such small items give us great satisfaction.

Almonds

Hazelnuts

Pecans

Pumpkin seeds

Sesame seeds

Sunflower seeds

Walnuts

WHAT TO DRINK

A quick word on fluids. While herbal teas, roasted-grain coffees, and kukicha tea are all great beverages to enjoy along with the occasional fruit or vegetable juice, beer, or wine with dinner, remember that there is only one fluid that truly hydrates us, water. All these other choices, while delicious and enjoyable, are simply luxuries and, in fact, in the case of teas, can actually dry us out a bit.

If you find that you are always thirsty, rather than just drinking more, check out your diet. Perhaps you are consuming too much sweet or salty tastes, both of which can trigger strong thirst.

NEED MORE?

Still feeling like a change to a healthy eating plan is a grim and deprived way to eat and that your life is over, culinarily speaking? Well, I'm in awe of the sheer volume of variety available to us. But if this isn't enough for you, remember that there's also variety in cooking styles and cutting techniques.

Even with all the variety that nature provides, if you're steaming everything and seasoning consists of a sprinkle of lemon juice, you'll grow bored, imbalanced in your nutrition and life energy, and your glow will falter. From roasting and baking to sautéing to frying to boiling, blanching, and yes, even steaming, cooking styles offer us variety and influence the quality of our foods and how we feel eating them.

From dicing to matchsticks to large chunks to slicing to grating and mincing, the preparation of your ingredients for cooking will influence how they taste and their visual appeal.

Remember that the kitchen is a place of nourishment and love. Cooking is an artistic expression of the passion of life that exists in all of us. To nourish others and ourselves is the most divine of art forms and to be considered anything less sells it, and us, short.

SO WHAT DO YOU DO NOW?

Now that we have all this variety, ingredients, seasonality, cooking, and cutting styles, how do you create a menu? Here's a framework to help guide you in your own menu plans.

Breakfast

Just like your mother told you, this is the most important meal of the day. This is the meal that sets the tone of your day. Will you be calm and graceful? Will you ride an emotional roller coaster? This meal is breaking the fast you have been on throughout the night as you slept. Your digestion needs a gentle nudge into action, just as you need a gentle nudge to awaken. Soft foods that are easy to digest are the true breakfasts of champions.

While you may enjoy the delicious flavor of fruit, remember that fruit has high concentrations of simple sugars and starting your day with fruit sets you up for blood chemistry chaos, with sugar "highs" and the crashes that follow.

The breakfast I recommend may take some getting used to, but once you get over the idea of soup and vegetables before noon, you'll find that you sail through your morning right to the lunch hour.

A light miso soup, with a small piece of wakame (for minerals) and few pieces of finely cut vegetables makes an energizing start to the day. Opening and relaxing the digestive tract, miso soup readies us for the day. Remember to keep it simple and vary the vegetables.

With miso soup, I like to serve a soft grain porridge that has the texture of oatmeal but is made from any variety of grain, both whole and cracked. Combining grains or using them on their own, with or without vegetables and sometimes with fruit, these porridge recipes are simple to create. Using five parts water to one part grain and cooked until the grain is soft and creamy, porridge is a delicious start to the day.

Finally, I like boiled, blanched, or steamed greens with breakfast. It may seem strange, but give it a try. Eating greens in the morning lifts our spirits and refreshes our energy, so that we begin the day feeling light and energized.

On special occasions or on those days when time is not so abundant, we'll enjoy some whole-grain bread and spreads or whole-grain pancakes or waffles with cooked fruit.

And once again, nothing's written in stone here. If you don't want soup every morning, take a risk and skip it. Or have a light breakfast of lightly cooked greens and soft bread. You decide which combination of foods makes you feel and look your best to get through the morning.

Lunch

To keep life simple, lunch can consist of leftover food from last night's dinner. If that's too abundant, try a bowl of soup with a side dish of cooked vegetables or a chunk of whole-grain bread. Occasionally, finish off lunch with a fresh salad or a piece of seasonal fruit and you have the perfect light meal.

Dinner

Okay, here's the challenge, I know. We live in a world that leaves us little time to passionately cook with abandon, creating feasts for our families to enjoy. And it's been to our detriment. Yes, I am asking that you return to the kitchen and cook, and it will be work. You may have to re-prioritize your day to allow for the kitchen time you need, but you will feel better, have more energy, and look like you've taken to napping.

Depending on your lifestyle and eating patterns, dinner can be a multi-dish feast or a one-pot supper. As long as you vary the ingredients, cutting styles, and cooking techniques, you'll see the difference.

Dinner in my house varies. On most nights, we begin with a soup course. Soup should set the tone for the meal. A simple soup should precede a hearty meal, while a hearty soup can be the leadoff for a simple meal. Bean soups take the place of a protein dish in the meal, so you can create a simple dinner when making a bean soup. Our main meal consists of a grain dish, a protein source (unless I make a bean soup), and two vegetable side dishes, usually, a light pickle for digestion, and because I like it, there's always a simple dessert. On other nights, we might have noodles with vegetables, lightly sautéed and served with greens, or polenta with a vegetable and bean ragout spooned over the top, again with lightly cooked greens or a fresh salad on the side. The only consistent thread among my evening meals is that they are rich in several vegetables to keep us well nourished and interested.

THE PLAN

Finally, we get to the plan. Here's what average menu plans might look like in my own house. You'll notice a lack of specific recipe titles. My goal here is simply to provide a framework that shows you how to create balanced menu plans for you. Fill them in as you desire to fit your own needs and taste.

BREAKFAST
Miso soup with vegetables
Soft-grain porridge
Boiled leafy greens

■
Lightly steamed bread with natural preserves
Blanched leafy greens
Tea

■
Whole-grain pancakes or waffles with cooked seasonal fruit
Tea

■
Soft-grain porridge
Scrambled tofu
Lightly steamed greens

LUNCH
Vegetable, grain and veggie, or bean and veggie soup
Whole-grain bread
Lightly cooked vegetables

■
Whole-grain sandwich of humus, baked tofu, and grilled vegetables with lettuce
Leftovers from dinner

DINNER
Soup
Grain, pasta, or cracked grain

Beans, tofu, or tempeh

Vegetable dish

> **Root veggie sauté**
>
> **Vegetable stew**
>
> **Boiled salad with dressing**
>
> **Oven-roasted vegetables**
>
> **Sea vegetables**

Lightly cooked leafy greens

Dessert

I recommend you get started by sitting down with the recipes you want to try and writing out some menu plans for yourself. You'll see if you're making too many dishes, too many complicated recipes, too many simple recipes, too much of any one ingredient (are there carrots in every dish or three protein sources?). You'll see what the meal will be like before you create it and you'll have an efficient shopping list to work from. After a couple of weeks of this kind of planning, you'll find that your intuition takes over and you simply shop and cook, creating simple, elegant, balanced meals.

YOUR GLOWING LIFESTYLE

We live in a world where it is quite difficult to maintain a natural balance. Everything around us pushes us to work harder, make more money, and move more quickly. Even our leisure time is frenetic with activity; we go on a holiday, only to come home exhausted and broke, from sightseeing and shopping.

Most of us live or work in less than natural surroundings, in many cases, in high-rise buildings without open windows, breathing stale, recycled air, which creates a stagnant atmosphere. Encased in this environment, we are surrounded by computers, fax machines, copiers, fluorescent lights, and other devices that take us farther and farther from nature. Surrounded by "white noise," we grow exhausted.

Think about how you feel when you take a holiday to a beach or camping. Out in nature, moving to the natural rhythms of your surroundings, your body changes. You wake early in the day with no alarm. You eat at regular intervals and find that you aren't binging and snacking throughout the day. By returning to natural surroundings and rhythms, the body is allowed to shift into a more natural way of being. It's the reason that even a weekend away, with no agenda, is so incredibly refreshing. If we observe nature, we will notice that she is wiser than us. She maintains periods of activity and periods of rest, in perfect balance.

I am not suggesting that we all vacate our lives, move to the country, and accomplish nothing. I am suggesting, instead, that we strive for a bit of balance, that we take care of ourselves so that we can accomplish our goals and realize our dreams.

With a few simple adjustments to our lifestyle and our own environment, we can create a space where we live more in balance with nature.

HOW TO EAT

As important as what we eat, is how we eat; it is the key to achieving and maintaining our ideal weight.

Whenever I travel in Europe, I am struck by the differences in the eating patterns I see around me. In America, we consume large portions and will eat anytime, anywhere, while walking, driving, working, as though eating were an intrusion on our busy lives. In Europe, especially Italy and France, meals are an event, a time in the day to be savored as much as the food itself.

In America, we're often confused by the fact that we are so much more conscious of fat and cholesterol and whatever else, and yet, we grow more obese—even our children. And in Europe, where they seem to eat with abandon, they remain (overall) more slender. There are reasons. One is that they sit down to eat, whether it's a meal or snack. They sit and eat; digestion is eased and they are less likely to eat without thought. Second, the portions in their meals are more reasonable, more normal for weight maintenance. Here in the United States, we want huge portions, more for our money, and we pay the price. If your portions are downsized, your food choices are sensible, and you eat in a more relaxed manner, you will achieve the weight you desire.

A FEW MORE POINTERS ABOUT EATING

1. Chew your food until it is liquid in your mouth. Unless you chew well, digestion is overworked, and we grow exhausted as we struggle to digest and utilize the nutrients in our food.

2. Eat only when really hungry. Try not to eat when bored or upset or tense. When we eat only when we are hungry, our body gets a break from working. We also eat a bit less. That, coupled with not exhausting our digestion with poor choices, goes a long way toward achieving our ideal weight.

3. Sit down when you eat. When sitting, the stomach softens and opens, creating a "belly," so that we can receive and utilize food more efficiently. Avoid eating while walking and driving; it's indigestion and overeating just waiting to happen.

4. Eat until you're satisfied, but not "Thanksgiving full." Remember that it takes the body twenty minutes to register that it has been fed. If you eat slowly, you'll be satisfied with less volume and not feel bloated.

5. Avoid eating for two to three hours before going to bed. If you eat before bed, the body spends much of your valuable rest time working to digest your midnight snack. You wake up feeling less than refreshed and begin your day tired, and the downward spiral of exhaustion continues.

6. Try to eat at the same time every day, in regular intervals. The body likes ritual and habit and knowing when you'll eat next helps you to eat less and keep digestion efficient and smooth. Eating at regular intervals also helps to prevent so much snacking. Decide how long you can go between meals and schedule accordingly, even if it means several small meals in place of three larger ones.

A bit of natural balance goes a long way in keeping us vital.

1. Try to retire before midnight and rise early in the day for the most restful sleep.

2. Try to get outdoors each day, regardless of the weather. It keeps us in touch with nature and stimulates us with natural energy from the earth, air, and sun.

3. Keep your home environment clean and orderly. Orderly surroundings make us feel more calm and safe, while a chaotic home agitates our frazzled nerves.

4. As much as possible utilize natural materials in your home, like cotton sheets, pillowcases, and towels, incandescent (rather than fluorescent) lighting, and natural carpeting and flooring. Use stainless steel, earthenware, or cast-iron cookware. Avoid aluminum and nonstick pots and pans for your cooking. Bring nature into every aspect of your life.

5. Open the windows every day, if possible. Even just a crack in a window or two for ten to fifteen minutes each day will freshen and enliven the air in your home, particularly in the bedroom, where we need to be refreshed with the best possible air to face our challenging days.

6. Place several green plants throughout your home. They freshen the air in our surroundings and enrich the oxygen content of the air we breathe.

7. If you work on a computer, keep a green plant close by to enrich the oxygen content of the air. Plants will also help you to stay a bit more hydrated, as computers make us feel dry and tired.

8. Take a break. If you are working at a desk or at a computer, take a stretch break for about ten minutes every hour or two. This will prevent tight back muscles and stiff joints, refocus your energy, and keep you from feeling exhausted.

EXERCISE

The importance of exercise in our lives is without measure. When we move our bodies, we improve circulation; our skin releases toxins; our muscles work and grow strong; our bones hold their density; we burn away our excess; and here's the best part, we feel great. Our mood improves; our self-esteem increases. It's hard to remain cranky when you step out the door into the sunshine and walk for thirty minutes or open a window and pull out the yoga mat and stretch your powerful muscles for fifteen minutes. We breathe deeply, drawing essential oxygen into our bodies, clearing our heads and allowing us to think. We walk taller and straighter; we have beautiful skin and a better attitude.

Exercise causes the heart to beat faster, which makes it more efficient and, in the long run, allows it to rest more often. Exercise lowers blood pressure by opening veins and arteries and improving circulation. Exercise increases our body's demand for fuel, burning stored calories and body fat. Exercise strengthens the bones by increasing bone growth and mass and by strengthening muscles, reducing stress on the bones.

So what should you do? I could advise you to try a few regimes and see what you like, and that's okay. I think, though, that you have to look at your life and how you live, and what you want to achieve. For exercise to work for you, it has to feel natural for you to do it. If you live life at a frantic place, "running" all the time, perhaps running is not the sport for you. Maybe yoga or tai chi or a dance class would feel more balanced to you. Rather than pushing yourself, even in exercise, you can choose a sport that helps to soften your edges, while keeping you fit.

If, on the other hand, you are a bit more sedentary in your work, then go for a walk or take up running or power yoga, something to get your juices flowing, again making balance for your less than active day.

There's no such thing as no time for exercise. It's as simple as walking to the grocery store or post office instead of driving. Walk a few flights of stairs, instead of taking the elevator all the way to the office. Take a walk at lunchtime, or walk to work or to the train station. Scrub floors by hand, in place of the mop, for a great upper body workout. Mow the lawn on foot and keep the tractor in the garage once in awhile.

There is no more natural exercise for us than walking. Human beings are built to walk. Walking is a blessing, our most natural form of motion. Don't think of it as exercise. Think of it as a gift to your body. With your legs pumping and arms swinging and drawing in breaths, you are working the circulatory and respiratory systems, heart, and muscles, and it doesn't even feel like exercise. There's no expensive equipment, no gyms, no pressure. A thirty-minute walk can make a world of difference in your body and your attitude.

Exercise at least three days a week, but five times is best to achieve your best overall health and for your radiant glow to really shine.

YOUR GLOWING ATTITUDE

How we feel about life and not just our own little world says a lot about us. People with giving hearts and gratitude for life seem more beautiful to us. They glow with vitality because they realize that there is more to life than our little place in it.

We all need to redevelop our appreciation of nature. Each day as you move through the world take a moment to marvel at the wonders of the world around you, from the vastness of the sky to the simplest wildflower sprouting through the cracks in the sidewalk. It's time to regain your sense of wonder at the miracle of life.

Try to live each day happily, regardless of personal struggles and challenges. Life is never smooth; you can either cave under the pressure or find your strength of character in challenge.

Be grateful for your life and all that it entails, even your difficulties. Show gratitude for the many blessings you have—family, friends, neighbors, life and work, the food you eat. Each day, each breath we take is a blessing for which we must be deeply grateful.

Begin to see your life, work, tasks, chores, and relationships as an important part in creating a healthy and peaceful world. Community and neighborhood work, help and care for the sick and lonely, providing comfort for those who suffer, all these things help us to see that we are one family and that working together, we can create a better world to live in. People who give of themselves are radiant with the fulfillment they receive from sharing, more than any cosmetic or even healthy food can ever provide. To look your best, join the human race.

SELF-CARE

This is an important aspect of our health and overall well-being, which results in whether or not we look our best. From the cosmetics we use to the water we drink, from rest and relaxation to moving our energy, there are simple steps we can take to allow our body to relax and naturally shift into its most balanced state.

Life is complicated. Most of us are busier than we ever dreamed we would be, with responsibility piled on responsibility. I won't add to your burden here, but taking care of yourself is the only way that you'll have the strength to step up to the plate each day. No matter how busy, we all need a few minutes to ourselves, to nourish our souls and be just a tiny bit indulgent. These commitments to our health help us sail through the day, feeling more relaxed and looking great.

Self-Care Pointers

1. As much as possible, avoid the use of chemical cosmetic products, from shampoo to hand cream to foundation and mascara. Look for products containing natural ingredients. Our body has no idea how to process unnatural chemicals and wears itself down. Remember that our skin absorbs whatever is put on it into our body. Those chemicals leach into our system and exhaust us.

2. And while we're on the subject of makeup and such, always, always, always wash your face before sleeping. No matter where you are or how tired you might be, take five minutes and cleanse your skin before bed. The skin needs that rest time during the night to discharge toxins and absorb moisture, so you wake up looking refreshed instead of tired and puffy.

3. When washing your face, take the time to rinse your face with cool water at least twenty times. This rids the skin of dead cells and prevents bacteria from forming on the surface of the skin.

4. In the morning, if you have cleaned your face properly the night before, you'll only need to rinse with cool water, again twenty times, to freshen your skin and rinse away any toxins discharged

naturally during sleep. If you wash with soap in the morning, you can dry your skin.

5. Massage your puffy eyes away. Starting at the inside corners of your eyes and using your index finger, press firmly at the lower, inside corner, applying pressure for 30 to 45 seconds. Then move to the outer corner of the eye and press firmly, again for 30 to 45 seconds. Next, press the depression between the top of the bridge of the nose and the upper corner of the eyes, again, for 30 to 45 seconds. Finally, move to the depression at the outer tip of the eyebrow and press firmly for 30 to 45 seconds. Repeat the whole massage twice.

6. Have a natural face-lift. Sit in a quiet place and breathe deeply. Begin by rubbing cheeks up and down until warm. Place hands over closed eyes and breathe deeply several times. Using two fingers, press gently but firmly around eye sockets, moving from inside to outside and around. Repeat several times. With two fingers, press the fronts of the eyeballs. Quickly detach and repeat several times. Use the thumb and index finger to pinch the bridge of the nose at the corners of the eyes. Press deeply for several seconds. Release and repeat several times. Rub up and down the sides of the nose until it feels warm. Using two fingers on each hand, massage the upper lip, from under the nose, working around the periphery of the mouth. Repeat ten times. Place thumbs underneath cheekbones and massage area for several seconds in a circular motion. Press thumbs under lower jaw, beneath ears. Repeat three to five times. Press around ear several times and end up by pulling ears in all directions twice. Finally, massage temples with two fingers in a circular motion for several seconds.

7. Rid your brow of those annoying little frown lines between the eyebrows. Find the spot above the center of each eyebrow that is one thumb-width above the brow. Using your index finger, press firmly into this spot for 30 to 45 seconds. Release pressure and repeat.

8. To rid your body of temporary fluid retention, try this simple shiatsu technique. Working with first your left leg and then the

right, follow this sequence. Find the spot three thumb-widths below the kneecap, to the outside of the tibia (shin bone). Press firmly for 30 to 45 seconds. Next, move to the spot on the inside of the calf, three thumb-widths up from the anklebone, and press firmly for 30 to 45 seconds. Next, move to the spot just below the inside of the knee at the head of the shin and press firmly for 30 to 45 seconds. Finally, move to the soft spot just below the inside anklebone and press firmly for 30 to 45 seconds. Repeat this sequence on the right leg.

9. The best, and the most important, is the body scrub. Do the body scrub every day without exception, or at least as often as humanly possible. The more often you scrub your skin, the quicker you'll see the results, from soft, satinlike skin to fewer pimples, to loss of water weight (see The Body Scrub, page 313).

Finally, use the scrubs, potions, brews, scalp massage, and skin treatments from Remedies to Glow By (pages 307–19) as you might need, to reclaim, and maintain, your glow.

Recipes

Sexy Soups

You may not think of soup when you think of beauty treatments, but you should. Soup is the most amazing food. The starter course to the meal, soup sets the tone for the rest of the feast that will follow, or it can be the feast itself.

So what's up with soup? Why all the fuss about this simple food? Soup's effect in the body is quite profound, especially in how we look and feel. Setting the tone for the meal is only the beginning. Soup, in fact, is largely responsible for how well we digest the meal we eat. Try an experiment. Begin dinner with soup one day and without, the next. Really observe the difference in how you assimilated the food you consumed on each day. Were you hungry an hour after dinner or did you remain sated all evening?

Soup works in the body to effectively draw energy and warmth into the digestive tract, relaxing and stimulating its function, so that when you take in solid foods, the process of digestion is already at work. When the body can digest food easily, it's less stressed. The work of digestion is smoother, more efficient. Two things occur. The body doesn't work so hard to nourish itself, and the body is satisfied with less food, because when digestion is more efficient, you are nourished more completely, with less volume.

Soup is also like a golden elixir for our skin and hair. Being a warm liquid, soup has an energy that draws moisture and nutrition deep into the body, particularly to the intestines. So the ingredients of the soup, using the liquid as the vehicle, travel deep into the body carrying the nutrients, but more important, the energy of the vegetables, grains, or beans to the intestines, liver, and kidneys efficiently and quickly. When these three organs are working well, they come together in a symphony of energy influencing the quality of our blood, making it strong and clean, which in turn, nourishes the skin and hair and nails to be their best.

Here's how it works. If you want skin that is less oily and prone to break-outs, you might choose to make a soup with daikon and shiitake mushrooms, both of which are reputed to work in the body to break down and eliminate accumulated fat which can result in common skin problems. If your problem is dry, tight skin, you might choose to sauté your vegetables before cooking them in soup to add the richness of oil to the pot, to soften the dryness. You might also choose vegetables with a sweet, moist nature, like winter squash, onions, dark leafy greens and green cabbage.

So make a fresh pot of soup every day. Savor its deep nourishment and delicious energy—and watch as a more youthful and beautiful—and sexier you is created with each spoonful.

Vegetable Miso Soup

Miso is the world's best-kept beauty secret. Rich in calcium, protein, vitamin D, and, most importantly, friendly bacteria (which aid in the production of digestive enzymes), miso is our most powerful anti-aging weapon. It strengthens our ability to assimilate food and take nourishment from what we eat, which in turn nourishes our skin, hair, and nails to be their best. ■ MAKES 4 SERVINGS

> 4-inch piece wakame, soaked until soft, finely diced
>
> 4 cups spring or filtered water
>
> ½ yellow onion, cut in thin, half-moon slices
>
> 1 small carrot, cut in thin coins
>
> ½ cup finely shredded green cabbage
>
> 2 teaspoons barley or brown rice miso
>
> 2 to 3 scallions, thinly sliced on the diagonal, for garnish

Combine the wakame and water in a saucepan. Cover and bring to a boil. Add the remaining vegetables, cover, and return to a boil. Reduce heat to low and simmer until the vegetables are soft, 5 to 10 minutes. Remove a small amount of broth, use to dissolve the miso, and stir back into soup. Simmer, uncovered, 3 to 4 minutes to activate the enzymes. Serve garnished with sliced scallions.

Clear Broth with Daikon

Daikon should be classified as the eighth wonder of the world. With a fresh, peppery taste, it's versatile and delicious. But its ability to help the body to break down, assimilate, and get rid of excess fat and protein makes it dear to our hearts. When the blood is free of build-up, the flow through the veins and arteries is smooth and efficient, creating a glowing complexion, strong, shiny hair, and vibrant energy. ■ MAKES 4 SERVINGS

4 cups spring or filtered water

4-inch piece kombu, soaked until soft, thinly sliced

4 button mushrooms, brushed free of dirt, thinly sliced

4 (½-inch) daikon rounds

Soy sauce

2 to 3 scallions, thinly sliced on the diagonal, for garnish

Bring the water and kombu, covered, to a boil. Add the mushrooms, cover, and return to a boil. Meanwhile, score the daikon rounds in a crisscross pattern to allow the thick slices to cook quickly. Add the daikon to the soup, cover, and simmer over low heat until daikon is tender, but not mushy, about 10 minutes. Season to taste with soy sauce and simmer 5 minutes more. Serve garnished with sliced scallions.

Winter Squash and Millet Soup

This deliciously sweet soup will relax the middle organs of the body: the spleen, pancreas, and stomach. And your looks? Think about how great your face looks after a relaxing vacation, ten years younger. Removing constricting stress from the body will relax the face and open the body so you can breathe more deeply, oxygenating the blood and creating a smooth, relaxed, youthful face.

■ MAKES 6 TO 8 SERVINGS

1-inch piece kombu

1 yellow onion, finely diced

2 stalks celery, finely diced

1 cup finely diced winter squash (butternut, buttercup, kabocha)

½ cup yellow millet, rinsed well

5 to 6 cups spring or filtered water

2 to 3 teaspoons white miso

2 to 3 scallions, thinly sliced on the diagonal, for garnish

Layer the kombu, onion, celery, squash, and millet in a soup pot. Gently add water, cover, and bring to a boil. Reduce heat to low and simmer soup until vegetables are tender and millet is creamy, about 35 minutes. Remove a small amount of broth, use to dissolve the miso, and stir back into soup. Simmer, uncovered, 3 to 4 minutes to activate the enzymes. Serve garnished with scallions.

Spicy Carrot Soup with Asian-Style Greens

This soup is so delicious, it'll take your breath away. Sweetly strengthening carrots will ground and center you, stimulating hot spices will increase circulation, and the lightly sautéed greens will create healthy red blood cells. You'll have beautiful, clear eyes, smooth circulation, and strong blood that will keep you looking and feeling your best. ■ MAKES 6 TO 8 SERVINGS

½ teaspoon hot chile sesame oil

1 teaspoon light sesame oil

1-inch piece fresh ginger, grated, juice extracted

1 yellow onion, diced

Sea salt

½ cup red lentils, rinsed well

6 to 8 carrots, diced

6 cups spring or filtered water

2½ teaspoons white miso

ASIAN-STYLE GREENS

½ teaspoon light sesame oil

2 scallions, cut into 1-inch pieces

½ cup mung bean sprouts

1 bunch watercress, cut into bite-size pieces

Soy sauce

Heat the hot and light sesame oil in a soup pot and add the ginger juice. Add the onion and a pinch of salt and sauté until translucent, about 2 minutes. Stir in the lentils and carrots and sauté until coated with oil, about 2 minutes. Add the water, cover, and bring to a boil over medium heat. Reduce heat to low and simmer the soup until the carrots are tender and the lentils are creamy, about 35 minutes. Transfer the soup, by ladles, through a chinois or food mill to create a smooth puree. Return to the soup pot. Remove a small amount of broth, use to dissolve the miso, and stir back into soup. Simmer, uncovered, 3 to 4 minutes to activate the enzymes.

While the miso simmers, prepare the greens: Heat the sesame oil in a small skillet and lightly sauté the scallions and mung bean sprouts to coat with oil, about 30 seconds. Stir in the watercress and season lightly with soy sauce. Sauté just until watercress wilts, about 2 minutes.

Serve the soup in individual bowls, with a hearty garnish of sautéed greens.

Sweet Adzuki Soup

There's nothing quite like azuki beans to take ten years off your face. Most of us begin to show our age when the delicate skin around the eyes grows puffy or develops dark circles and creases. Those common symptoms are a sign that the kidneys are overtaxed and tired, growing weak and flaccid. These little red beans help to rebalance the kidney function, restoring the youthful appearance of our eyes. ▪ MAKES 6 TO 8 SERVINGS

> 1-inch piece kombu
>
> ½ cup adzuki beans, rinsed well, soaked for 4 hours
>
> 5 to 6 cups spring or filtered water
>
> 1 small leek, split lengthwise, rinsed well, thinly sliced
>
> 1 carrot, diced
>
> 1 cup diced winter squash (butternut, buttercup, kabocha)
>
> 1 cup finely diced green cabbage
>
> 3 teaspoons barley or brown rice miso
>
> 2 to 3 leaves kale, finely diced, for garnish

Place the kombu on the bottom of a soup pot. Top with the beans and water. Bring to a boil, uncovered. Cook for 5 minutes over medium heat. Cover, reduce heat to low, and simmer for 35 minutes. Add the vegetables, cover, and cook until the beans are soft and the vegetables are tender, about 35 minutes more. Remove a small amount of broth, use to dissolve the miso, and stir back into soup. Simmer, uncovered, 3 to 4 minutes to activate the enzymes. Stir in the kale and serve.

Sweet Corn and Butternut Squash Soup

The combination of sweet corn and winter squash is as natural as summer turning to autumn. The corn nourishes our heart and circulatory system, and the sweetness of the squash enhances the function of the spleen, stomach, and pancreas. That means clear skin, strong hair, and a line-free, relaxed face, with a healthy blush to the cheeks. ▪ MAKES 6 TO 8 SERVINGS

2 small butternut squash, halved lengthwise, seeds removed

Light olive oil

Sea salt

6 to 7 cups plain soy milk

1 onion, diced

2 cups fresh or frozen corn kernels

1 tablespoon mirin

½ teaspoon powdered ginger

½ teaspoon ground cinnamon

2½ teaspoons white miso

2 to 3 scallions, thinly sliced on the diagonal, for garnish

Preheat the oven to 400F (205C) and lightly oil a shallow baking dish. Oil the squash halves, covering the entire surface. Sprinkle the cut sides lightly with salt. Arrange in baking dish, cut-side down, cover loosely, and bake until the squash is quite soft, about 45 minutes.

When the squash is cooked, scoop the flesh from the squash halves and place in a soup pot with the soy milk. Add a pinch of sea salt, cover, and bring to a boil. Reduce heat to low and simmer 10 minutes. By ladles, put the soup through a chinois or food mill to create a smooth puree. Return to the soup pot and add the onion, corn kernels, and spices. Bring to a boil, covered, over medium heat. Reduce heat to low and simmer until onions are tender, about 10 minutes. Remove a small amount of broth, use to dissolve the miso, and stir back into soup. Simmer, uncovered, 3 to 4 minutes to activate the enzymes. (Thin the soup with a little water if needed.) Serve garnished with scallion slices.

Fresh Corn Soup

Ever look at a corn kernel, really look at one? Notice the plump, flawless complexion on each kernel. Smooth, line-free skin—our heart's desire. We spend billions on the quest. Fresh summer corn nourishes our skin to be its best by stimulating circulation and the function of the small intestine, making for supple, flawless skin of our very own. ■ MAKES 4 TO 6 SERVINGS

> **2 tablespoons light olive oil**
>
> **1 yellow onion, diced**
>
> **Sea salt**
>
> **7 to 8 ears fresh corn, kernels removed**
>
> **3 cups plain rice milk or soy milk**
>
> **1 teaspoon white miso**
>
> **3 to 4 fresh chives, minced, for garnish**
>
> **1 red bell pepper, roasted over an open flame, peeled, seeded, minced (see below), for garnish**

Heat the oil in a soup pot over medium heat. Add the onion and sauté with a pinch of salt 1 to 2 minutes. Stir in the corn and rice milk, cover, and bring to a boil over medium heat. Reduce heat to low and simmer for 15 to 18 minutes. Remove a small amount of broth, use to dissolve the miso, and stir back into soup. Simmer, uncovered, 3 to 4 minutes to activate the enzymes. Transfer the soup to a food processor and puree until smooth (the soup will be thick). Return to soup pot and simmer, uncovered, 1 to 2 minutes. Serve soup garnished with a sprinkle of chives and roasted peppers.

NOTE To roast a bell pepper, rinse and dry the pepper and place over an open flame. Cook, turning, with tongs, until the outer skin of the pepper is completely charred. Transfer the pepper to a paper sack, seal, and allow the pepper to steam for about 10 minutes. Gently rub the charred skin from the pepper and rinse gently to remove any charred residue. Roasted peppers will keep, refrigerated, for about a week.

Bread and Cabbage Soup

A traditional Italian stew, this soup is so delicious, eating it makes you look better instantly. Seriously, ever notice the lovely skin common to most Italian people? A lot of their beauty comes from their diet, especially the use of olive oil and fresh vegetables. The cabbage at the center of this soup has the unique ability to nourish and relax the middle organs of the body: the spleen, pancreas, and stomach, leaving the face looking fresh and relaxed. ▪ MAKES 6 TO 8 SERVINGS

About 4 tablespoons extra-virgin olive oil

1 onion, diced

Sea salt

1 pound green cabbage, diced

Generous pinch dried basil

2 tablespoons mirin

5 to 6 cups spring or filtered water

2½ teaspoons barley or brown rice miso

6 to 8 thick slices whole-grain sourdough bread

Small bunch flat-leaf parsley, minced, for garnish

Heat about 2 tablespoons oil in a soup pot over medium heat. Add the onion and sauté with a pinch of salt, about 2 minutes. Stir in the cabbage, sprinkle with salt and basil, and sauté until the cabbage begins to wilt, about 3 minutes. Add the mirin and water, cover, and bring to a boil over medium heat. Reduce heat to low and simmer until vegetables are quite soft, about 25 minutes.

While the soup cooks, preheat oven to 375F (190C). Brush the bread slices generously with oil and place on a baking sheet. Bake, uncovered, until the bread is lightly browned and toasted.

Remove a small amount of broth, use to dissolve the miso, and stir back into soup. Simmer, uncovered, 3 to 4 minutes to activate the enzymes.

Stir parsley into soup just before serving. There are two options for serving: You can place a slice of bread in individual bowls, spoon soup over top, and serve. You may also layer bread with soup in a large tureen and scoop individual servings of bread and soup into bowls.

White Bean and Vegetable Soup

Bringing together beans and sweet root vegetables makes us feel strong and vital, a sure way to look your best. But it doesn't end there. This potent combination, by strengthening our digestive system, makes for strong, thick, lustrous hair.

■ MAKES 6 TO 8 SERVINGS

> **1-inch piece kombu**
>
> **1 small leek, split lengthwise, rinsed well, thinly sliced**
>
> **1 small rutabaga, diced**
>
> **1 to 2 parsnips, diced**
>
> **2 to 3 carrots, diced**
>
> **2 to 3 stalks celery, diced**
>
> **1 cup Great Northern or white navy beans, rinsed well and soaked 2 hours**
>
> **6 cups spring or filtered water**
>
> **3 teaspoons white miso**
>
> **2 to 3 fresh scallions, thinly sliced on the diagonal, for garnish**

Lay the kombu on the bottom of a soup pot and layer the vegetables on top, in the order listed. Top with drained beans and gently add water. Cover soup and bring to a boil over medium heat. Reduce heat to low and simmer until beans are soft, about 45 minutes to 1 hour. Remove a small amount of broth, use to dissolve the miso, and stir back into soup. Simmer, uncovered, 3 to 4 minutes to activate the enzymes. Serve garnished with sliced scallions.

Sweet Parsnip Soup with Hazelnut Pesto

There's nothing quite as beautifying as sweet, creamy soups. Relaxing to the middle organs—spleen, pancreas, and stomach—great for strengthening digestion, a rich bisque-like soup is like the fountain of youth. The smooth, creamy consistency of the soup is easy to digest, supporting, rather than exhausting, digestive function, which helps to strengthen the blood to nourish our skin to be line-free and flawless and our hair shiny and strong. ■ MAKES 6 TO 8 SERVINGS

1 onion, diced

1 small leek, split lengthwise, rinsed well, diced

6 to 8 parsnips, diced

3 cups plain rice milk or soy milk

3 cups spring or filtered water

¼ cup mirin

2½ teaspoons white miso

Small bunch fresh flat-leaf parsley, minced, for garnish

HAZELNUT PESTO

1 cup hazelnuts, oven-toasted, skinned (see Note, below)

1 cup loosely packed fresh basil leaves

1 cup loosely packed fresh flat-leaf parsley

3 shallots, diced

¾ cup extra-virgin olive oil

2 teaspoons white miso

2 teaspoons umeboshi vinegar or fresh lemon juice

1 teaspoon brown rice syrup

Layer vegetables in a soup pot in the order listed. Gently add rice or soy milk, water, and mirin. Cover and bring to a boil over medium heat. Reduce heat to low and simmer until parsnips are quite soft, about 30 minutes. Remove a small amount of broth, use to dissolve the miso, and stir back into soup. Simmer, uncovered, 3 to 4 minutes to activate the enzymes.

While the soup cooks, make the pesto: Combine all ingredients in a food processor and puree until smooth. You will have more pesto than you may need for this recipe. It will keep, refrigerated, for about a week.

Transfer soup, by ladles, through a chinois or food mill to create a smooth puree. Return to pot and simmer for 1 minute. Serve, garnished with a generous dollop of pesto and sprinkled with minced parsley.

NOTE To roast hazelnuts, arrange nuts on a baking sheet and bake at 325F (165C) for 15 to 20 minutes, until fragrant. Transfer nuts to a paper sack and allow skins to loosen in the steam for about 10 minutes. Then rub nuts in a towel to remove the skins.

Shiitake and Black Soybean Soup

Black soybeans have long held the reputation for supporting reproductive function, being rich in phytoestrogens, calcium, vitamin D, and protein so essential to health. Combining them in a rich, flavorful broth with shiitake mushrooms, which are reputed to aid the body in breaking down accumulated fat, makes for a soup that will leave your skin even-toned and glowing, with no pimples around the mouth or on the chin, nor wrinkles, dimples, lines, and creases in the chin area, indicators that our reproductive organs are overworked and sluggish.

■ MAKES 6 TO 8 SERVINGS

1 cup black soybeans (see Note below), sorted

1-inch piece kombu

9 cups spring or filtered water

2 teaspoons light sesame oil

1 yellow onion, diced

Sea salt

1 carrot, diced

1 cup diced daikon

1 cup diced green cabbage

4 to 5 dried shiitake mushrooms, soaked until soft, thinly sliced

2 tablespoons mirin (optional)

2½ teaspoons barley or brown rice miso

2 to 3 fresh scallions, thinly sliced on the diagonal, for garnish

Rinse, drain, and towel-dry the soybeans to remove any excess water, so they will toast evenly. Heat a dry skillet and add soybeans. Dry-roast over medium heat until the beans puff and the skins begin to split, about 10 minutes. Transfer beans to a pressure cooker. Work kombu to the bottom of the pot with a chopstick or spoon handle, add 3 cups of the water, and bring to a boil, uncovered. Allow to boil for 5 minutes. Seal pressure cooker lid and bring to full pressure. Reduce heat to low and cook beans for 40 minutes. Remove pot from heat and allow pressure to reduce naturally. Drain beans.

Heat the oil in a soup pot over medium heat. Add the onion and sauté with a pinch of salt until limp, about 2 minutes. Add the carrot, daikon, and a pinch of salt and sauté for 1 minute. Stir in the cabbage and a pinch of salt and sauté until shiny with oil. Stir in the mushrooms and sprinkle with mirin if using.

Add cooked beans and remaining 6 cups of water. Cover and bring to a boil over medium heat. Reduce heat to low and cook soup until vegetables and beans are quite soft, about 25 minutes. Remove a small amount of broth, use to dissolve the miso, and stir back into soup. Simmer, uncovered, 3 to 4 minutes to activate the enzymes. Serve garnished with sliced scallions.

NOTE You may use canned organic black soybeans in this recipe to make a quicker cooking soup, but the flavor will not be as full nor will you receive the full vitality of the beans.

Spring Greens Soup

There's nothing quite like spring to let you know that you have a liver; you can grow easily irritated, for instance. More telling, though, are those deep little furrows between your brows; we know them as frown lines. They are telling us that our liver is overworked and aggravated. A soup like this one, with calming grains and laced through with astringent bitter greens, will refresh your energy, open the liver, and relax those lines, and your temper. ■ MAKES 6 TO 8 SERVINGS

Spring or filtered water

1 red onion, diced

Sea salt

1 small leek, split lengthwise, rinsed well, and thinly sliced

1 cup diced daikon

½ cup white basmati rice (do not rinse)

2½ teaspoons white miso

4 to 5 leaves fresh basil, shredded

6 to 7 stalks broccoli rabe, dandelion, or mustard greens or 1 small bunch
    watercress, rinsed, shredded

2 to 3 scallions, thinly sliced on the diagonal, for garnish

Heat about 2 tablespoons water in a soup pot over medium heat. Add onion and water-sauté with a pinch of salt, until limp, about 2 minutes. Stir in the leek and a pinch of salt and cook 1 minute. Stir in the daikon and rice and cook 1 minute. Add 5 to 6 cups water, cover, and bring to a boil over medium heat. Reduce heat to low and simmer until rice is quite creamy, about 25 minutes. Remove a small amount of broth and use to dissolve the miso. Stir into soup with basil and broccoli rabe. Simmer 3 to 4 minutes to cook broccoli rabe and to activate the enzymes of the miso. Serve garnished with scallions.

Sweet Vidalia Soup with Cornmeal Toasts

There's nothing as sweetly relaxing as onion soup. Richly sautéed, sweet Vidalia onions are the basis for this beauty of a first course. Think of onions and then think skin. Onions are richly moist, smooth, and plump. Their sharp taste cleanses our bodies of accumulated fat, allowing moisture to seep into the skin, making it beautifully smooth. ▪ MAKES 8 TO 10 SERVINGS; ABOUT 24 CORNMEAL TOASTS

1 tablespoon extra-virgin olive oil

8 to 10 Vidalia onions, thinly sliced into half-moon pieces

Sea salt

1 tablespoon mirin

6 cups spring or filtered water or vegetable stock

Soy sauce

2 to 3 fresh scallions, thinly sliced on the diagonal, for garnish

CORNMEAL TOASTS

½ cup yellow cornmeal

¼ cup whole-wheat pastry flour

¼ teaspoon sea salt

½ teaspoon baking powder

1 tablespoon light olive oil

½ cup spring or filtered water

Heat the oil in a soup pot over medium heat. Add the onions and sauté with 2 to 3 pinches of salt until they begin to wilt. Stir in the mirin and reduce heat to medium-low. Continue to cook, stirring frequently, until onions reduce and begin to caramelize, about 20 minutes. They should be nicely browned. Slowly add the water to just cover onions, and bring to a boil. Reduce heat to low, add the remaining water, cover, and simmer for 20 minutes. Season to taste with soy sauce (lightly, remember the soup is to be sweet) and simmer 5 to 7 minutes more to develop the flavors.

To make the toasts: preheat oven to 375F (190C) and line 1 or 2 baking sheets with parchment paper. Combine the cornmeal, flour, salt, and baking powder. With a pastry cutter or fork, cut in the oil to create the texture of wet sand. Stir in enough water to make a stiff dough. Transfer dough to a pastry bag fitted with a ¼-inch fluted tip. Pipe the dough into 3-inch-long strips onto the baking sheets, leaving about 1 inch between them. Bake until the strips are crisp and golden and curl just a bit, about 10 minutes.

To serve the soup, spoon into individual bowls, garnished with scallions and several cornmeal toasts.

Gorgeous Grains

Whole cereal grains are the foundation of health, the centerpiece food for humanity. So is it any wonder that grain would be an essential factor in how you look day to day?

We all know that the fiber in whole grains is an important factor in the prevention of colon cancer, diverticulitis, ulcers, appendicitis, hemorrhoids, and many other digestive disorders, but we really don't associate digestive function with good or bad hair days. Well, we should. The health, and therefore, appearance, of our hair depends largely on the functioning of the microvilli in the small intestine. The quality of nutrients taken into the body, along with how well they are assimilated, is responsible for nourishment or starvation of the hair follicles. Therefore, foods that strengthen digestion and stimulate circulation are essential for a head of strong, lustrous hair.

The soluble fiber found in grain, especially brown rice and oats, has been found to lower cholesterol, reducing the risk of coronary diseases, but also preventing blockages in capillaries that supply nutrients to the hair follicles.

Because of their structure, the complex carbohydrates in whole grains are also essential to beautiful hair. Since they break down slowly, they are not absorbed as quickly. So unlike simple carbohydrates (sugars) that are rapidly absorbed, complex carbohydrates will strengthen the ability of the digestive system to circulate nutrients to the hair.

Whole grains also contain perfectly balanced nutrients—an average of seven to one, which matches the ratio between active growth and rest periods of the hair growth cycle. In whole grains, the ratio of minerals to protein is about one to seven; protein to carbohydrate is also one to seven, making grain the ideal food to support and nourish smooth, even growth cycles of the hair.

But whole grains do more than give us that magazine-model hair we all desire. The fiber, complex sugars, minerals, protein, and B vitamins so abundant in them nourish our skin as well. The intestines are responsible for regulating moisture in the body as well as for influencing the quality of the blood that will nourish all of our organs, determining their health and function. If the intestines are able to do their job properly, then we don't look puffy under the eyes, washed out, or pale. Conversely, if moisture is properly balanced, we won't be plagued by dry skin, tightness on the face, or little lines and wrinkles that come from dryness. If the intestines are efficiently nourished, their work influences the creation of strong, balanced blood, which in turn circulates through our other organ systems, creating flawless skin, even color, and very few problems in the way of blemishes or other imperfections.

So go to the kitchen and cook a pot of rice; you'll forget hot oil treatments, leave-in conditioners, and the zillions of other products we use to simulate the appearance of great skin and hair. Within days, your skin will glow with health and quickly take on that flawless appearance we all covet. It may take a few months to see the difference in your hair, since it needs to grow out to be visibly different, but you will finally have the hair and skin that seem to live only in commercials.

Gomoku

This splendid rice stew is a traditional Asian dish designed to create vitality. The ingredients come together to cleanse the blood of accumulated fat and protein that make for sluggish organ function. And when various organ systems are working together in harmony, the blood that nourishes the skin and hair is clean and strong, so you look and feel your best. ■ MAKES 3 TO 4 SERVINGS

1-inch piece kombu

1 cup short-grain brown rice, rinsed well

½ yellow onion, finely diced

1 small carrot, finely diced

2 dried shiitake mushrooms, soaked until tender, finely diced

2 to 3 slices dried lotus root, soaked until tender, finely diced

¼ cup dried shredded daikon, soaked until tender, finely diced

Soy sauce

2 cups spring or filtered water

1 teaspoon fresh ginger juice

1 to 2 scallions, thinly sliced on the diagonal, for garnish

Place the kombu on the bottom of a pressure cooker. Top with the rice and layer the vegetables over the rice in the order listed. Season lightly with soy sauce and gently add water, taking care not to disturb the layering too much. Seal the lid and bring to full pressure over medium heat. Place the pot on a flame deflector, reduce heat to low, and cook for 50 minutes. Remove from heat and allow pressure to reduce naturally. Open the pot, stir ginger juice gently into ingredients to combine, and transfer to a serving bowl. Serve garnished with scallions.

Ruby Rice

Bringing together two powerhouses of moisture regulation, short-grain brown rice and adzuki beans, ensures that we look our best. Brown rice is the most incredible moisture-balancing agent in nature. If you're retaining water, rice will help to absorb and dispel it. Feeling parched, with dry skin and hair? Brown rice will help the body hold the liquid it needs. Azuki beans, little red, jewel-like beans, provide us with protein and potassium and are low in fat. Reputed in Asia to be restorative of kidney function, azuki beans aid in getting rid of dark circles under the eyes by keeping the kidneys soft and working efficiently and you looking fresh and alert.

■ MAKES 4 TO 5 SERVINGS

> ½ cup adzuki beans, sorted, rinsed, soaked for 4 hours
>
> 2 cups spring or filtered water
>
> 1 cup short-grain brown rice, rinsed well
>
> 1-inch piece kombu

Drain the beans and place in a small saucepan with 1 cup of the water. Bring to a boil over medium heat and cook for 5 minutes.

Place the rice, remaining 1 cup water, azuki beans, and cooking water in a pressure cooker. Push the kombu to the bottom of the pot with your finger or a spoon handle. Seal the lid and bring to full pressure over medium heat. Reduce heat to low, place pot on a flame deflector, and cook for 50 minutes. Remove from heat and allow pressure to reduce naturally. Stir gently to combine and transfer to a serving bowl. Serve hot or warm.

Sweet Brown Rice with Black Soybeans

This rich grain dish makes the most beautiful hair. Black soybeans, rich in protein and minerals like calcium, are reputed to be restorative to the reproductive and digestive systems, helping to create healthy intestinal flora. Combining that with the higher protein content of sweet brown rice makes this a powerhouse of vitality. ■ MAKES 4 TO 5 SERVINGS

> ½ cup black soybeans, sorted
>
> 1 cup sweet brown rice, rinsed well
>
> 2 cups spring or filtered water
>
> Soy sauce
>
> 1 to 2 scallions, sliced thinly on the diagonal, for garnish

Rinse, drain, and towel-dry the soybeans to remove any excess water, so they will toast evenly. Heat a dry skillet and add soybeans. Dry-roast over medium heat until the beans puff and the skins begin to split, about 10 minutes. When 80 percent of the beans have split, they are done. Do not over-roast or the beans will burn.

Place the rice, roasted soybeans, and water in a pressure cooker. Cover loosely and bring to a boil. Add a dash of soy sauce and seal lid. Bring to full pressure over medium heat. Reduce heat to low, place pot on a flame deflector, and cook for 50 minutes. Remove from heat and allow pressure to reduce naturally. Open pot and stir ingredients gently to combine. Transfer to a serving bowl and serve garnished with scallions.

Asian-Style Basmati Rice

Basmati rice has a light, fresh energy, and aromatic flavor that lifts our spirits and makes us look and feel wonderful, especially when the weather is hot and sticky, leaving you feeling and looking limp. Cooked with lightly sautéed vegetables, this grain dish brings out the sparkle in your personality. You'll look fresh and feel charming. ▪ MAKES 4 TO 5 SERVINGS

1 tablespoon toasted sesame oil

1 yellow onion, diced

Soy sauce

1 carrot, diced

1 cup diced daikon

1 to 2 stalks celery, diced

1½ cups brown basmati rice, rinsed well

2 cups spring or filtered water

1 cup finely shredded kale or collard greens

Heat the oil in a heavy pot over medium heat. Add the onion and a dash of soy sauce and sauté until limp, about 2 minutes. Stir in the carrot, daikon, and a dash of soy sauce and sauté 1 minute. Add the celery and cook until just shiny with oil. Spread the vegetables evenly on the bottom of the pot. Top with the rice and gently add the water. Cover and bring to a boil over medium heat. Season lightly with soy sauce, cover, and reduce heat to low. Cook until rice has absorbed all the liquid, 45 to 50 minutes. Remove cover and stir the kale gently into rice to combine. Serve hot or warm.

Sautéed Corn with Ginger and Scallions

Who doesn't want clear, sparkling eyes that dance with mischief? You can have them with this dish. Fresh, sweet corn is infused with the fiery energy of summer, which in turn creates a sparkling vitality in us. Ginger is a strong root that works deep in the body to stimulate circulation, and when your blood is pumping efficiently, there's a healthy glow to your skin that can't be found in any compact.

■ MAKES 3 TO 4 SERVINGS

> 2 teaspoons light olive oil
>
> 5 to 6 slices fresh ginger, cut into fine matchstick pieces
>
> 2 cups fresh corn kernels
>
> Soy sauce
>
> 5 to 6 scallions, cut into ½-inch pieces
>
> 3 to 4 stalks broccoli rabe, rinsed well, thinly sliced
>
> ½ red bell pepper, roasted over an open flame, peeled, seeded, sliced into
>> thin ribbons (see Note, page 178)

Heat the oil in a skillet or wok over medium heat. Add the ginger and sauté for 1 minute. Stir in the corn and add a dash of soy sauce and sauté 1 minute. Add the scallions and a dash of soy sauce and sauté for 1 minute. Stir in the broccoli rabe, season lightly with soy sauce, and sauté until the broccoli rabe wilts and turns a deep green, about 3 minutes. Transfer to a serving platter and serve garnished with the bell pepper.

Polenta with Roasted Vegetables

Creamy soft cornmeal topped with richly roasted vegetables and succulent mushrooms. Sound like heaven? It should. It'll make you look heavenly as well. I love how this dish works. With polenta, you have creamy texture, which relaxes the body, but since it's corn, it is infused with sunny summer energy, making you feel vital. The sweet vegetables come together to nourish the middle organs, relaxing any tension. And the mushrooms are quite supportive of kidney function, making them work efficiently and smoothly. Our face is relaxed and line-free, with not a puffy bag or dark circle in sight.

■ MAKES 6 TO 8 SERVINGS

POLENTA

5 cups spring or filtered water

Dash soy sauce

1 cup yellow corn grits

Generous pinch dried basil

ROASTED VEGETABLES AND PORTOBELLOS

1 red onion, cut into thin half-moon slices

¼ head green cabbage, cut into 1-inch chunks

1 cup 1-inch pieces winter squash (red kuri or buttercup is best)

1 carrot, cut into 1-inch irregular pieces

2 portobello mushrooms, stems removed, quartered

About 3 tablespoons extra-virgin olive oil

About 2 teaspoons soy sauce

About 2 teaspoons balsamic vinegar

Grated zest of 1 lemon

Juice of ⅓ lemon

Parsley sprigs, for garnish

To prepare the polenta: Place all the ingredients in a saucepan and whisk to combine. Bring to a boil over medium–low heat, whisking frequently to prevent lumping and scorching. Reduce heat to low and cook polenta over low heat, whisking frequently, until the center of the polenta bursts, like a big bubble. (Caution: the bubbles can splatter and cause burns.) Spoon the polenta evenly into a lightly oiled shallow baking dish and set aside. The polenta will be firm after about 30 minutes.

While the polenta cooks, prepare the vegetables: Preheat the oven to 350F (175C). Combine the vegetables in a large mixing bowl and drizzle generously with olive oil, season lightly with soy sauce and balsamic vinegar, and sprinkle with the lemon zest. Toss gently to combine and spread vegetables evenly in a shallow baking dish or pie plate.

Cover and bake for 35 minutes. Remove cover and bake for another 20 minutes, or until the vegetables are soft and beginning to brown. Remove from oven and sprinkle with the lemon juice.

To serve, slice the polenta into squares or wedges. Place the polenta on a plate and spoon a generous amount of roasted vegetables over top. Garnish with a few parsley sprigs.

Carrot-Parsnip Risotto

The strengthening character of root vegetables comes together with the relaxing energy of Arborio rice to create a dish that will turn your hair into your crowning glory. This delicious dish uses the energy of the root vegetables to draw the rich moisture of the dish deep into the body to create soft, lustrous hair. The quality of our hair is determined by the condition of our intestines. With root vegetables' natural tendencies to strengthen intestinal fortitude, they work to create a strong, shiny mane. ▪ MAKES 3 TO 4 SERVINGS

5 cups spring or filtered water

3 tablespoons extra-virgin olive oil

1 red onion, diced

Sea salt

2 to 3 parsnips, finely diced

2 to 3 carrots, finely diced

1 cup Arborio rice (do not rinse)

¼ cup mirin

Small bunch flat-leaf parsley, finely minced, for garnish

Place the water in a saucepan over low heat. Keep it warm throughout the cooking process.

Heat the oil in a deep skillet over medium heat. Add the onion and a pinch of salt and sauté until limp, about 2 minutes. Stir in the parsnips and carrots and sauté until shiny with oil, about 1 minute. Stir in the rice and mirin. Cook, stirring frequently, until the liquid is absorbed into the rice. Add additional water, by ½-cup ladles, stirring frequently, only as it is absorbed into the dish. The finished risotto will cook in about 30 minutes total cooking time and will be creamy, but the rice should retain some firmness. Stir in minced parsley and serve immediately.

Millet "Fries" with Glazed Carrots

Millet has the ability to relax any tension in the body by nourishing the energy of the spleen, pancreas, and stomach. Millet is the only whole grain that produces no stomach acid and so is quite easy to digest.

In this recipe, we sauté leftover millet sticks to create a rich, crispy crust. Serve smothered in succulent, sweet carrots and you have a dish that deeply relaxes the body, regulates blood chemistry, and gives you skin that is smooth, supple, evenly toned, and line-free. ■ MAKES 5 TO 6 SERVINGS

MILLET "FRIES"

1 cup cooked millet (see Note, page 196)

Yellow cornmeal

Light olive oil

GLAZED CARROTS

1 yellow onion, cut into thin half-moon slices

4 to 5 carrots, cut into 1-inch irregular pieces

Grated zest of 1 lemon

2 to 3 tablespoons brown rice syrup

Soy sauce

Juice of 1 lemon

To prepare the "fries": Press the cooked millet into a rectangular, shallow baking dish. It should be about ¼ inch thick. Set aside until firm, 30 to 35 minutes. When the millet is set, cut it into 3 × ¼-inch spears. Dredge each spear in cornmeal. Heat about ¼ inch oil in a deep skillet over medium heat. (Test it by submerging the tips of wooden chopsticks in the oil. If bubbles gather around the sticks, the oil is ready.) Add the millet sticks in batches and fry until golden, turning to brown evenly, 1 to 2 minutes on each side. Drain on paper towels. Continue frying until all the millet is used.

To make the carrots: Place the onion in a saucepan and top with the carrots, lemon zest, and rice syrup. Add a dash of soy sauce and gently pour in enough water to just cover the bottom of the pan. Cover and bring to a boil over medium heat. Reduce heat to low and simmer until carrots are quite soft and the cooking liquid has turned into a thin syrup. Remove from heat and gently stir in the lemon juice.

To serve, pile several "fries" on individual plates and smother with the carrots. Serve warm.

NOTE To cook millet for this recipe, place 1 cup millet, 4 cups spring or filtered water, and a pinch of salt in a saucepan. Bring to a boil, covered, over medium heat. Reduce heat to low and simmer until millet is creamy and liquid is absorbed into the grain, 30 to 35 minutes.

Hato Mugi with Roasted Corn and Shallots

Known as "beauty pearls" in Asia, hato mugi barley is prized for its ability to restore the complexion to flawless perfection. This mild-mannered grain works to cleanse the blood of accumulated fat that can make the skin look lifeless and washed out. Adding to the vitality of the dish is the sweet luxury of roasted corn and sweet shallots, which will add a bit of sparkle to our eyes and keep our faces stress-free. ■ MAKES 3 TO 4 SERVINGS

5 to 6 shallots, halved

2 ears fresh corn, husked

Extra-virgin olive oil

Soy sauce

About 1 tablespoon brown rice syrup

1 cup hato mugi barley, sorted, rinsed well

2 cups spring or filtered water

Small handful flat-leaf parsley, minced, for garnish

Preheat oven to 375F (190C). Lightly oil a shallow baking dish.

Lightly rub the shallots and corn with oil and soy sauce. Place in baking dish and drizzle lightly with rice syrup. Roast in the oven, uncovered, until the shallots are tender and browned and the corn has begun to brown, about 35 minutes, turning corn after 15 minutes to ensure even roasting. Remove from oven and cool enough to be able to touch the corn comfortably. When you can handle the corn, use a sharp knife and remove the kernels from the cobs and dice the shallots.

Place vegetables on the bottom of a pot and top with the hato mugi and water. Bring to a boil, loosely covered. Add a dash of soy sauce and cover. Reduce heat to low and cook until barley has softened and all the liquid has been absorbed, about 35 minutes. Remove from heat and stir in the parsley. Serve warm.

Sesame-Scallion Corn Muffins

I don't know anyone who can resist the temptation of muffins (at least not happily). Besides the pure enjoyment of eating them, these miniature beauties provide a special energy. Cornmeal, with its characteristic coarseness, helps the body to digest the flour, easing the process. The scallions provide a light, uplifting energy to prevent the heaviness often associated with flour products, and the sesame seeds provide vitality and calcium. The result is little, gemlike muffins that lift our spirits and leave us looking alive.

■ MAKES ABOUT 24 MINI MUFFINS OR 12 STANDARD MUFFINS

3 tablespoons light olive oil

1 bunch scallions, rinsed, finely diced

1 cup yellow cornmeal

1 cup whole-wheat pastry flour

2 teaspoons baking powder

⅛ teaspoon sea salt

¼ cup tan sesame seeds

¼ cup light olive oil

¼ cup brown rice syrup

½ to 1 cup plain soy milk

½ cup black sesame seeds, for garnish

Preheat oven to 350F (175C) and lightly oil a 24-cup miniature muffin pan or 12-cup standard muffin pan (you may also use foil liners).

Heat the oil in a skillet over medium heat. Add the scallions and sauté until bright green and limp, about 1 minute. Set aside to cool.

Combine the cornmeal, flour, baking powder, salt, and tan sesame seeds in a medium bowl. Mix in the oil and rice syrup to blend. Slowly stir in enough milk to make a thick, spoonable batter. Fold in the sautéed scallions.

Divide the batter evenly among muffin cups. Sprinkle with black sesame seeds. Bake until golden and firm to the touch, 20 to 30 minutes. Cool for about 10 minutes before carefully removing muffins from the pan. Serve warm or at room temperature.

Whole-Wheat Soda Bread

Ah, flour products, we love them, but do they serve us in maintaining our health and our looks? They can. White bread, white pasta, and white flour pastries can cause us to feel sluggish and stuck, with lifeless skin, dull, dry hair, and dry patches on our heels, knees, shins, and elbows. Whole-grain flour, on the other hand, can actually help to relax the body, allowing digestion to calm and work more efficiently. When digestion is smooth, the blood nourishing our skin and hair makes them look their best. ■ MAKES 1 LOAF

2 cups whole-wheat flour

1 cup whole-wheat pastry flour

½ cup rolled oats

2 teaspoons sea salt

2 teaspoons baking soda

2 teaspoons baking powder

1 cup plain rice milk or soy milk

⅛ cup umeboshi vinegar

⅛ cup brown rice syrup

⅛ cup light olive oil

Preheat oven to 350F (175C).

Combine the flours, oats, salt, baking soda, and baking powder, in a large mixing bowl. In a separate bowl, mix the milk and umeboshi vinegar together (this simulates a buttermilk flavor). Combine with the rice syrup and oil. Stir into flour mixture to create a sticky dough. On a lightly floured work surface, knead the bread until it's smooth, about 10 minutes.

Shape into a round loaf and transfer to an ungreased baking sheet or stone. Refine the shape, and using a sharp paring knife, cut a large cross shape in the top of the loaf (so it doesn't split as it rises).

Bake until the bread is golden brown and sounds hollow when tapped, 45 to 50 minutes.

VARIATION After shaping the loaf, brush lightly with olive oil and sprinkle with sesame seeds or crushed pumpkin seeds to add extra flavor, texture, and the vitality of the seeds.

Chinese Scallion Cakes with Dipping Sauce

A very traditional Asian-style bread, it is not baked in the oven but rather on a hot skillet. Baked flour can make digestion sluggish, leaving you feeling stagnant.

Cooked over open heat, rather than in the oven, and filled with peppery scallions, this light bread will relax the body, with the energy of the ginger and scallions improving circulation, making for a flawless complexion, with a touch of color in the cheeks. ■ MAKES 18 WEDGES

CHINESE SCALLION CAKES

2 cups whole-wheat pastry flour

1 teaspoon baking powder

½ teaspoon sea salt

2 tablespoons toasted sesame oil

¾ cup spring or filtered water

Brown rice flour

1 cup minced scallions

Light olive oil, for cooking

DIPPING SAUCE

1 cup spring or filtered water

1 tablespoon soy sauce

1 teaspoon brown rice vinegar

1 teaspoon fresh ginger juice (see Tip below)

Juice of ½ lemon

To prepare the cakes: Combine the pastry flour, baking powder, salt, and sesame oil, mixing well. Add water and mix until dough gathers into a ball. Transfer dough to a lightly floured surface and knead until silky, about 2 minutes. Cover with an inverted bowl and allow to rest for 1 hour.

Knead dough a couple of times to loosen. Dust surface of dough liberally with rice flour. Roll out dough to a 17-inch square about ⅛-inch thick. Sprinkle generously with scallions to cover the surface of the dough. Roll up, jelly-roll style, to form a firm cylinder. Cut into 3 equal portions. Roll each portion back and forth on the work surface to create a long rope. Coil the rope around itself to make a circular bread about an inch thick. Cover with plastic and repeat with other coils.

Dust work surface with more rice flour and roll each coil into a 9-inch circle. Scallion bits will break through the dough during rolling.

Lightly oil a griddle or cast-iron skillet and warm over medium-high heat. When a sprinkling of water dances across the surface, the skillet is hot enough. One at a time, cook the breads until lightly browned, 2 to 3 minutes on each side. Press any bubbles out of the breads with a metal spatula. Drain on paper towels and cover to keep warm, while cooking remaining breads.

To make the dipping sauce: Combine all ingredients in a small bowl.

Cut each cake into 6 wedges and serve warm, with the sauce on the side.

NOTE To extract juice from fresh ginger, grate unpeeled ginger root on a fine grater and squeeze pulp.

Wild Rice with Hato Mugi and Vegetables

Who doesn't want perfect skin, free of lines, spots, dots, pimples, or blemishes? Whole grains and vegetables promote efficient organ function, influencing the creation of strong blood and creating the flawless complexion we all crave.

■ MAKES 4 TO 5 SERVINGS

1 yellow onion, diced

1 cup diced fresh daikon

1 cup fresh or frozen corn kernels

1 to 2 stalks celery, diced

1 cup hato mugi barley, sorted, rinsed well

½ cup wild rice, rinsed well

3 cups spring or filtered water

Soy sauce

2 stalks broccoli, cut into small florets, stalks peeled and diced

In a pressure cooker, layer the onion, daikon, corn, and celery. Top with the barley and wild rice. Add the water, cover loosely, and bring to a boil over medium heat. Add a dash of soy sauce and seal the lid. Bring to full pressure, reduce heat to low, and place pot on a flame deflector. Cook for 35 minutes. Remove from heat and allow pressure to reduce naturally.

While the barley cooks, bring a small pot of water to a boil and cook broccoli until bright green and crisp-tender, about 4 minutes.

To serve, gently stir the broccoli through the cooked barley and vegetables to combine ingredients. Serve warm or chilled.

Chilled Soba with Lemony Asparagus Sauce

Buckwheat is the most amazing grain. Grown under adverse conditions, this hearty grain gives us strength and endurance that makes us stand tall and straight and walk with confidence.

The asparagus and lemon work together in this dish to deeply cleanse and relax the liver and gallbladder, those organs responsible for ridding the body of toxins that not only make the skin look dull and lifeless, and the whites of eyes less than white, but also create those irritating little furrows between our brows.

■ MAKES 3 TO 4 SERVINGS

> 1 pound fresh asparagus, ends snapped off, cut into 1-inch pieces
> 2 tablespoons extra-virgin olive oil
> Sea salt
> Grated zest of 1 lemon
> 1 cup plain soy milk
> 1 teaspoon kuzu, dissolved in 2 tablespoons cold water
> 8 ounces soba noodles
> Lemon wedges, for garnish

Separate the asparagus tips from the stems and set aside.

Heat the oil in a skillet over medium heat. Add the asparagus stems, a pinch of salt, and lemon zest and sauté until bright green and tender, about 2 minutes. Add the soy milk, season to taste with salt, and bring to a boil, covered, over low heat. Simmer for 5 minutes.

Transfer mixture to a food processor and puree until smooth. Return to the skillet and stir in reserved asparagus tips. Simmer over low heat until tips are bright green, about 2 minutes. Stir in dissolved kuzu and cook, stirring, until sauce thickens slightly.

While the sauce cooks, bring a pot of water to a boil. Add soba noodles and boil until tender, about 8 minutes. Drain and rinse well. (Japanese noodles are coated with salt during drying and require rinsing after cooking for the best flavor.)

To serve, toss noodles with asparagus sauce and serve warm, garnished with lemon wedges.

Soba Primavera

Buckwheat noodles are great for improving our intestinal fortitude, which in turn influences the quality of the blood created in our bone marrow, which in turn nourishes other organ systems, which in turn are reflected on our faces, as our skin is richly fed. Add the freshness and moisture of vegetables, which make our skin plump and supple, and you will revel in your glowing complexion.

■ MAKES 3 TO 4 SERVINGS

2 tablespoons extra-virgin olive oil

1 yellow onion, cut into thin half-moon pieces

Sea salt

½ teaspoon dried basil

1 carrot, cut into fine matchstick pieces

10 to 12 sun-dried tomatoes, soaked until soft, thinly sliced

2 cups small cauliflower florets

2 stalks broccoli, cut into small florets, stems peeled and thinly sliced

1 cup plain soy milk

1 teaspoon kuzu, dissolved in 2 tablespoons cold spring or filtered water

8 ounces soba noodles, cooked until tender, rinsed, drained well

Small handful flat-leaf parsley, minced, for garnish

½ red bell pepper, roasted over an open flame, peeled, seeded, diced (see
   Note, page 178)

Heat the oil in a deep skillet over medium heat. Add the onion, and a pinch of salt and basil, and sauté until limp, about 1 minute. Add the carrot, tomatoes, and a pinch of salt and sauté 1 minute. Add the cauliflower, broccoli, and a pinch of salt and sauté 1 minute. Add the soy milk, cover, and cook over low heat until broccoli is bright green and tender, 5 to 7 minutes. Season lightly with salt. Stir in the dissolved kuzu, and cook, stirring, until sauce thickens, about 3 minutes.

To serve, mound noodles on a platter and spoon vegetables and sauce over top. Garnish with minced parsley and bell pepper and serve immediately.

Orecchiette with Arugula Pesto

Bitter greens are the greatest thing for clarifying the skin. The bitter flavor and astringent quality cleanse the liver and gallbladder of any accumulated fat, which can interfere with the discharge of toxins. Bitter greens are also an important ingredient in the body's ability to digest, assimilate, and remove oil and fat. In this dish, we bring together the energy of bitter greens to tone the liver with the vitality and sweetness of nuts and oil to create a dish that will lift your energy, create clear skin with uniform color, clear whites of the eyes, and remove lines or wrinkles between the brows. ■ MAKES 5 TO 6 SERVINGS

ARUGULA PESTO

2 bunches arugula, stems removed, rinsed well, coarsely minced

1 bunch chives, rinsed well, coarsely minced

½ cup hazelnuts, roasted and peeled (see Note, page 181)

½ cup extra-virgin olive oil

2 teaspoons white miso

2 teaspoons brown rice syrup

2 teaspoons umeboshi vinegar

PASTA

1 pound orecchiette

1 red onion, cut into thin half-moon slices

Fresh chives, left whole, for garnish

To make the pesto: Bring a large pot of water to a boil and quickly blanch the arugula for about 30 seconds. Save this water to cook pasta. Combine the arugula and chives, transfer to a food processor, and pulse to puree. Add the hazelnuts, oil, miso, rice syrup, and vinegar. Puree until a thick smooth pesto forms. Set aside.

To cook the pasta: Return the water to a boil. Add the pasta and onion and boil until tender, 10 to 12 minutes. Drain, but do not rinse. Toss hot pasta with pesto to coat. Transfer to a serving bowl and arrange chives in a crisscross pattern on top of the noodles to garnish. Serve warm or chilled.

Penne with Roasted Vegetable Sauce and Olives

Sometimes it's hard to imagine that food that tastes deliciously decadent can be good for you. Here's a dish that will blast that myth to smithereens. Mild-mannered pasta provides the perfect opportunity for richly roasted root vegetables to come together with skin-enhancing olives to create a dish that will leave our complexion glowing with health. ▪ MAKES 3 TO 4 SERVINGS

¼ cup extra-virgin olive oil

2 teaspoons soy sauce

2 tablespoons balsamic vinegar

2 yellow onions, finely diced

3 to 4 carrots, finely diced

3 to 4 parsnips, finely diced

Spring or filtered water, as needed

3 to 4 leaves kale or collard greens, trimmed, left whole

1 pound penne pasta

1 cup oil-cured black olives, pitted, coarsely minced

Preheat oven to 350F (175C). Combine the oil, soy sauce, and vinegar in a small saucepan and warm over low heat 3 to 4 minutes. Arrange the onions, carrots, and parsnips in a shallow baking dish, avoiding overlap, and pour sauce over top to coat vegetables. Cover and bake for about 35 minutes. Remove cover, return to the oven, and cook about 15 minutes, or until the vegetables are soft and just beginning to brown. Do not overbrown or the sauce will be a dark, unappealing color.

Transfer the roasted vegetables to a food processor, and puree until smooth. Spoon sauce into a saucepan and warm over low heat, adding water to thin sauce to desired consistency.

Bring a large pot of water to a boil and cook the kale, just until bright green, about 2 minutes. Drain and slice into bite-size pieces. In the same water, cook pasta until tender, but still firm, 8 to 10 minutes. Drain pasta, but do not rinse.

To serve, toss cooked pasta with pureed vegetable sauce, kale, and olives. Serve warm.

Cavatelli with Roasted Squash Pesto

No one makes pasta quite like the Italians. Their passion for food, pasta in particular, makes for some of the lustiest recipes around. What's that got to do with your looks? Think Sophia Loren. One of her most famous lines was that she credited her looks to spaghetti.

In this recipe, we bring the sweetly flavored energy of baked winter squash together with moisture-rich onions to form a pesto-style sauce that will leave your face relaxed and line-free (as it calms and opens the middle organs, spleen, pancreas, and stomach). ■ MAKES 4 TO 5 SERVINGS

2 yellow onions, cut into thick half-moon slices

1 medium butternut squash, peeled, seeded, cut into 1-inch pieces

Sea salt

1 teaspoon dried basil

About 2 tablespoons barley malt

About 2 tablespoons mirin

1 cup lightly toasted sunflower seeds

¼ to ½ cup plain soy milk

1 pound cavatelli pasta

Small handful flat-leaf parsley, finely minced, for garnish

Preheat oven to 350F (175C). Combine the onions and squash in a shallow baking dish. Sprinkle lightly with salt and basil. Drizzle generously with barley malt and mirin. Cover and bake for 35 minutes. Remove cover and bake about 15 minutes, or until vegetables are quite soft and just beginning to brown.

Transfer roasted vegetables to a food processor. Add sunflower seeds and soy milk. Puree until smooth, adding more soy milk for a thinner consistency. (Don't thin too much; pesto sauces are best when kept thicker, as they will coat the pasta more effectively.) Transfer pesto to a saucepan and keep warm over very low heat while cooking pasta.

Bring a large pot of water to a boil and cook cavatelli until tender, but not mushy, 10 to 12 minutes. They will sink in the water and then rise to the top when they are close to done. Drain well, but do not rinse. Transfer to a serving bowl and immediately spoon squash pesto over top. Mix well to coat and serve immediately, garnished with parsley.

Soba with Shiitake Mushrooms and Scallions

Bringing together strengthening and calming energy creates serene endurance within us. In this dish, we combine the hearty character of buckwheat noodles with the relaxed energy of shiitake mushrooms, which will go deep into the body, especially effective in releasing any accumulated congestion in the kidneys. Stagnant kidneys make for puffy eyes and dark circles. Efficient kidneys make for clear skin, with no need of concealers. ▪ MAKES 3 TO 4 SERVINGS

2 tablespoons toasted sesame oil

1 yellow onion, cut into thin half-moon slices

½-inch piece fresh ginger, cut into fine matchstick pieces

Soy sauce

1 tablespoon brown rice syrup

1 carrot, cut into fine matchstick pieces

1 cup fine matchstick daikon pieces

6 to 8 dried shiitake mushrooms, soaked until soft, stems removed, thinly
sliced

1 small zucchini, cut into fine matchstick pieces

2 tablespoons mirin

1 cup spring or filtered water

1 cup shredded watercress

3 to 4 scallions, thinly sliced on the diagonal

1 teaspoon kuzu, dissolved in 2 tablespoons cold spring or filtered water

1 to 2 tablespoons umeboshi vinegar

8 ounces soba noodles, cooked until tender, rinsed, and drained well

Several slices pickled ginger, minced, for garnish

½ cup black sesame seeds, lightly pan-toasted, for garnish

Heat the oil in a wok over medium heat. Add the onion and ginger and sauté with a dash of soy sauce and the rice syrup until limp, about 1 minute. Stir in the carrot and daikon, add a dash of soy sauce, and sauté for 1 minute. Stir in mushrooms, zucchini, a dash of soy sauce, and the mirin. Add the water, cover, and cook over low heat until the mushrooms are tender, about 10 minutes. Stir in the watercress, scallions, and dissolved kuzu, and cook, stirring, until a thin glaze forms over the vegetables. Remove from heat and stir in the vinegar.

To serve, mound noodles on a platter and spoon vegetables over top. Garnish with pickled ginger and sesame seeds and serve immediately.

Udon with Dandelion Greens and Fava Beans

With whole-grain noodles as the base, sharp-flavored dandelion greens are easily digested and can do their job quite effectively, helping the liver to rid the body of excess or accumulated toxins. The buttery rich fava beans create the perfect balance for the astringent quality of the greens, making sure your moisture stays as the toxins leave. The result is beautiful, moist, plump, supple skin, free of those annoying little wrinkles between your brows that let you know your liver is tired.

■ MAKES 3 TO 4 SERVINGS

8 to 10 ounces dried fava beans, soaked 6 to 8 hours

4 to 5 cups spring or filtered water

1-inch piece kombu

1 yellow onion, diced

About 3 tablespoons extra-virgin olive oil

1 leek, split lengthwise, rinsed well, thinly sliced on the diagonal

Soy sauce

1 carrot, cut into fine matchstick pieces

2 to 3 bunches dandelion greens, rinsed well, sliced into 1-inch pieces

1 tablespoon mirin

8 ounces udon noodles

2 to 3 scallions, thinly sliced on the diagonal, for garnish

Drain soaking water from fava beans and place the beans in a saucepan. Add the spring water, kombu, onion, and 2 teaspoons olive oil. Bring to a boil, uncovered, and cook over high heat for 5 minutes. Reduce heat to low, cover, and cook until beans are just tender, 1 to 1½ hours. Drain liquid from beans and set beans aside.

Heat about 2 tablespoons olive oil in a deep skillet over medium heat. Add the leek and sauté with a dash of soy sauce until limp, about 2 minutes. Stir in the carrot, add a dash of soy sauce, and sauté 1 minute. Stir in the dandelion greens and mirin and season lightly with soy sauce. Sauté the greens until limp, but retaining a deep green color, about 3 minutes. Stir in the fava beans, cover, and keep warm on low heat until noodles are cooked.

Bring a large pot of water to a boil and cook the noodles until tender, 8 to 10 minutes. Drain and rinse well. (Japanese noodles are coated with salt during the drying process and require rinsing for the best flavor.) To serve, stir beans, greens, and any remaining cooking liquid with noodles to combine. Garnish with scallions.

VARIATION You can use 1½ pounds fresh fava beans in season, popping them from their pods, and then blanching the beans to remove the skins. Cook them with the dandelion greens mixture.

NOTE When using dandelion greens, try to find the organic version, because those you might harvest from the park, or even your own yard, will most likely contain pesticides.

Voluptuous Vegetables

Walking into a supermarket tells us all we need to know about the beauty found in nature. The first section of the market to greet you is fresh produce, abundantly stacked and artfully arranged. Think of how many times you've walked through aisles of fruits and vegetables, so struck by the beauty and vitality surrounding you, that you bought everything in sight, knowing full well that most of it would rot in the crisper drawer because you couldn't use it. But at that moment, overcome with the freshness, the color, the variety, you just *had* to have it.

The word "vegetable" comes from the Latin verb *vegetus*, meaning "lively, vigorous, fresh." When you walk into a beautiful produce section, you are struck, of course, by the vibrant colors, but what you are *really* attracted to is the sheer magnetism of life, of nature in its freshest, purest state. You identify with the living energy. To be surrounded by fresh, living vegetables makes us feel alive and vital. If you can see the beauty of nature, and you are what you eat, as I contend, well, you can figure it out. Vegetables are great beauty food.

Fresh vegetables are enlivened by the combination of the energies of the sun, earth, water, and air, creating a balanced vitality essential for life. Without vegetables in our diet, we grow weak. Disconnected from nature's life-giving energy, we find ourselves lost, searching for ways to strengthen and enliven ourselves. We take supplements, energy drinks, vitality bars; we ingest pills, take shots, and concoct potions on the quest for energy and vitality and eternal youth and beauty.

Vegetables give us so much energy, so much life. Vegetables, the original source of protein, give us protein in its purest form. You can eat vegetables and go directly to the source of the strength, avoiding the middle man, or middle cow. Vegetables are the best source of vitamins, minerals, and other nutrients. From folic acid to vitamin E to useable calcium to any other nutrient you can imagine (except vitamin B-12), you'll find them, in abundance, in vegetables. We need the nutrients that we get from vegetables, but I am much more enchanted by the incredible energy we get from fresh vegetables.

The vitality of life and beauty that we all crave so deeply is within easy grasp, in the humble bins of any farmers' market, natural-food store, or supermarket. To take your nutrients from the food you eat, instead of from pills, drinks, or other supplements (except where absolutely necessary), brings more to your body than just vitamin C, folic acid, and iron. You get to ingest the nutrients, of course, but more important, you merge with the energy of nature, the sun, the earth, the water, and the air. You reconnect with nature, nourishing yourself the way we nourish our beautiful plants and flowers, with energy and vitality. . . and life.

ROOT VEGETABLES

Look at root vegetables. They drill into the soil, drawing nutrients into their deep roots. They are firmly lodged in the ground; they know exactly where they are going. Including them in our diet brings similar energy into the body. Eating root vegetables, carrots, parsnips, turnips, rutabaga, daikon, and burdock, makes us stronger, influencing the quality of blood that nourishes the organs that, in turn, nourish the skin and hair.

GROUND VEGETABLES

The round, sweet vegetables that grow close to the ground include winter squash, head cabbage, onions, and Brussels sprouts. With their calm, quiet natures and delicious sweet flavors, these are the vegetables that help you keep your cool. Relaxing the middle organs, particularly the spleen and pancreas, helps the body to release toxins effectively and to regulate our blood sugar, preventing tense, tight muscles, stiff bones, and wrinkles on our faces.

GREENS

In my opinion, these leafy vegetables, including kale, collard greens, watercress, mustard greens, bok choy, broccoli rabe, dandelion, and arugula, are some of the most important foods we can consume to put our best face forward. Rich in antioxidants, calcium, vitamins C and D, iron, magnesium, and folic acid, these leaves may look delicate, but they are incredible sources of strength. Drawing nutrients completely into their leaves from their delicate roots means that the leaves are thoroughly nourished. Their rich green color is indicative of rich sources of chlorophyll and iron, which improves the strength of our red blood cells.

With dark leafy greens as a part of our daily diet, our faces remain line-free (because we handle stress well and because nutrients reach our faces efficiently), with perfect blemish-free, supple skin.

SEA PLANTS

Exotic sea plants are more than just unique. Rich in protein, calcium, vitamins, and minerals that enrich our skin, nails, and hair, these strong vegetables are essential to maintaining strong, well-balanced blood. Small amounts of these dense nutrients ensure that we nourish our organs (and thereby our faces) with essential nutrients for health. In my own experience, I know that I haven't seen a split end since adding these incredible vegetables to my diet.

So think veggies and have a beautiful day.

Lotus Root Kinpira

Kinpira is a classic Asian dish, meaning "golden pieces," designed to create vitality, strength, and focus. Using the strength of the burdock and carrot to draw the astringent properties of the lotus root deep into the intestines, we cleanse them of any accumulated congestion that can cause their function to become sluggish. When the intestines are clear of stagnant energy, the blood that nourishes the skin is clean and strong, making for a flawless, smooth complexion.

▓ MAKES 3 TO 4 SERVINGS

2 teaspoons toasted sesame oil

1 cup fine matchstick pieces burdock

Sea salt

1 cup fine matchstick pieces carrot

1 cup thin half-moon slices fresh lotus root

1-inch piece fresh ginger, grated, juice extracted (see Note, page 201)

Spring or filtered water

Soy sauce

¼ cup minced fresh flat-leaf parsley, for garnish

Heat the oil in a skillet over high heat. Add the burdock and sauté with a pinch of salt until shiny with oil, about 2 minutes. Spread the burdock evenly over the bottom of the skillet and top with the carrot, then lotus root. Sprinkle the ginger juice over top and add enough spring or filtered water to just cover burdock. Reduce heat to medium-low, cover, and cook for 10 minutes. Season lightly with soy sauce, cover, reduce heat to low, and cook until all liquid has been absorbed into the dish, about 7 minutes. Stir gently to combine and serve hot, garnished with minced parsley.

Roots and Tops

This is the perfect combination of light, fresh energy and rooted strength. Eating cooked root vegetables carries their energy deep into the body to create endurance and stamina. Stewing the root with the fresh, green tops creates a balanced energy that is unparalleled. While the root grounds us, maintaining strong blood, the green tops work to relax the body and to oxygenate the blood. Roots and tops relax hardened, overworked kidneys, helping us sleep soundly and get rid of those dark circles under our eyes. ■ MAKES 2 TO 3 SERVINGS

1 to 2 carrots, turnips, or small daikon, with tops
Soy sauce
¼ to ½ teaspoon chile powder
Spring or filtered water

Carefully remove the whole tops from the vegetable. Rinse well and set aside. Cut the roots of the vegetables into small, irregular pieces (about ¼ inch in size). Place roots in a saucepan with a dash of soy sauce and chile powder. Add enough water to half cover the vegetables. Cover and bring to a boil over medium heat. Reduce heat to low and simmer for 10 minutes.

While the roots simmer, finely mince the tops. Add the tops to the pot, season lightly with soy sauce, and simmer, covered, until the greens are just tender, but still bright green. Remove cover and increase heat to cook away any remaining liquid. Stir gently to combine and serve immediately.

Dried Daikon with Winter Squash

Daikon could easily be marketed as the greatest beauty product known to man, or woman. It possesses the uncanny ability to cleanse the body of stagnation that can make the organs' functions sluggish and leave us looking as stale as we feel. As a root vegetable, daikon travels deep into the body, with its peppery taste doing the cleanup. Dried daikon has had all its moisture removed, concentrating its cleansing properties, allowing it to travel even more deeply to cleanse and freshen various organ systems, creating glowing skin and a relaxed, line-free face.
■ MAKES 3 TO 4 SERVINGS

1 yellow onion, cut into thin half-moon slices

1 cup fine matchstick pieces winter squash (red kuri, butternut, or buttercup
   is best)

½ cup dried daikon, soaked until soft

Soy sauce

Spring or filtered water

Juice of 1 lemon

¼ cup minced fresh flat-leaf parsley, for garnish

Layer the onion, squash, and daikon in a saucepan. Add a dash of soy sauce and enough water to half cover the ingredients. Cover and bring to a boil over medium heat. Reduce heat to low and cook until vegetables are tender, about 40 minutes. Season lightly with soy sauce and simmer, covered, 7 to 10 minutes. Remove the cover and cook until any remaining liquid is absorbed into the dish. Remove from heat and stir in the lemon juice. Serve garnished with the parsley.

Sweet and Savory Carrots

Joining the natural sweet flavor of carrots with the briny, savory taste of black olives creates a dramatic dish and delicious energy in the body. Plump, supple olives help to create soft, moist skin, while the carrots draw energy and nutrients deep into the body to create strength and stamina. ■ MAKES 4 TO 5 SERVINGS

1 tablespoon extra-virgin olive oil

1 red onion, cut into ¼-inch-thick wedges

Sea salt

5 to 6 carrots, cut into 1-inch irregular chunk pieces

2 tablespoons capers, drained and lightly rinsed

2 teaspoons mirin

½ cup halved pitted black olives

¼ cup minced fresh flat-leaf parsley

Heat the oil in a skillet over medium heat. Add the onion and sauté with a pinch of salt until quite soft, about 4 minutes. Stir in the carrots and a pinch of salt and stir to coat with oil. Add the capers and mirin, cover, and reduce heat to low. Simmer, stirring occasionally, until the carrots are just tender, about 20 minutes. Season lightly with salt and stir in the olives. Simmer 2 to 3 minutes more. Stir in the parsley and serve hot or at room temperature.

Fresh Daikon and Scallion Salad

If this salad doesn't leave you looking clear-eyed and alert, nothing will. Bringing together the spicy, fresh taste of daikon and scallions will get your engine started. With daikon's unique ability to release congestion, scallions' ability to move energy up and out, and fresh lemon flavor to relax the liver, this dish helps to move stagnant energy, improves circulation, and creates flawless, glowing skin, lustrous hair, and strong, supple nails and vitality to burn, which is what really makes us look our best. ▪ MAKES 3 TO 4 SERVINGS

½ cup thin matchstick pieces carrot

2 cups thin matchstick pieces daikon

6 to 8 scallions, thinly sliced on the diagonal

3 to 4 tablespoons minced fresh flat-leaf parsley

LEMON DRESSING

2 tablespoons umeboshi vinegar

1 tablespoon brown rice vinegar

Juice of 1 lemon

1 tablespoon stone-ground mustard

2 tablespoons toasted sesame oil

2 teaspoons brown rice syrup

½ teaspoon soy sauce

2 to 3 leaves kale, steamed until tender

½ sheet toasted nori, shredded, for garnish

Bring a pot of water to a boil and blanch the carrot for 30 seconds. Remove with a slotted spoon and transfer to a mixing bowl. In the same water, blanch the daikon for about 1 minute. Drain and add to carrot. Mix in the scallions and parsley.

To make the dressing: Whisk dressing ingredients together in a small bowl. Adjust seasonings to taste. Toss the dressing with the vegetable mixture. To serve, line a plate with steamed kale, spoon salad on top, and mound shredded nori in the center.

Lemon-Scented Roasted Vegetables

We don't associate rich food with beauty, just the opposite. But a bit of richness in our diet, in the form of good-quality fat, nuts, and sweet flavors, relaxes the body, makes us feel satisfied, helps us to eat less (because we need less to feel sated) and that leaves our faces looking relaxed and youthful, line-free, soft, and clear, and our bodies, just the right size. ▪ MAKES 5 TO 6 SERVINGS

4 to 6 shallots, peeled, halved lengthwise

8 to 10 baby carrots

4 to 5 small parsnips, halved or quartered (depending on the size)

2 sweet potatoes, cut into 1-inch wedges

3 to 4 stalks celery, cut into 1-inch pieces

3 to 4 dried bay leaves

¼ cup hazelnuts

½ cup pecan halves

6 to 8 dried apricots, coarsely minced

2 to 3 tablespoons extra-virgin olive oil

Soy sauce

Grated zest of 2 lemons

Juice of 1 lemon

Parsley sprigs, for garnish

Preheat oven to 350F (175C). Lightly oil a large, shallow baking dish.

Combine the vegetables, bay leaves, nuts, and apricots in a mixing bowl and drizzle generously with olive oil. Turn gently to coat ingredients. Sprinkle lightly with soy sauce and add the lemon zest. Mix well to coat. Spread the vegetable mixture evenly in prepared baking dish.

Cover and bake about 40 minutes, or until tender. Remove cover and bake 10 to 15 minutes more, or until the vegetables are lightly browned. Remove from oven and toss with the lemon juice, taking care not to break the vegetables. Serve garnished with parsley sprigs.

Roasted Artichoke and Turnip Salad with Raspberry Vinaigrette

Artichokes can be quite wonderful for us on occasion. Their light energy and very specific growth pattern lifts our energy, while helping us to keep our focus. Combining them with sweet onions, sharp turnips, and a rich, delicately sweet dressing creates a symphony of flavors. This type of satisfying dish will help to relax the body, with the sumptuous dressing creating supple, plump, moisturized skin, and lustrous hair. ■ MAKES 4 TO 5 SERVINGS

1 pound small turnips, quartered

8 to 10 fresh artichoke hearts (see Note, page 220), halved lengthwise

2 red bell peppers, roasted over an open flame, peeled, seeded, quartered
  (see Note, page 178)

2 red onions, halved, each half cut into 4 wedges

3 to 4 tablespoons extra-virgin olive oil

About 1 tablespoon soy sauce

1 to 2 tablespoons balsamic vinegar

2 teaspoons fresh basil, finely minced

Grated zest of 1 lemon

1 bunch watercress, blanched

RASPBERRY VINAIGRETTE

2 tablespoons extra-virgin olive oil

2 teaspoons unsweetened raspberry preserves

½ teaspoon soy sauce

2 teaspoons stone-ground mustard

2 to 3 fresh scallions, finely minced

Preheat oven to 350F (175C). Bring a pot of water to a boil over medium heat. Add the turnips and cook 1 minute (to remove the bitter taste). Drain well and place in a mixing bowl. Stir in the artichoke hearts, bell peppers, and onions. Mix in a generous drizzle of oil and soy sauce and a light sprinkle of vinegar. Transfer vegetables to a large shallow baking dish and sprinkle with basil and lemon zest.

Cover and bake for 30 minutes. Remove cover, and bake 20 to 25 minutes, or until the vegetables are tender and browned.

While the vegetables roast, make the vinaigrette: Whisk all ingredients until well combined.

To serve, transfer roasted vegetables to a serving platter lined with blanched watercress, and drizzle generously with vinaigrette and serve warm.

NOTE To prepare an artichoke heart, cut the stem of the artichoke off at the base. Remove the outer leaves of the artichoke by pulling them down so they snap off. Using a sharp knife, cut the artichoke crosswise, removing most of the remaining leaves, leaving about a 1½-inch-thick base. With a small paring knife, trim the green leaf stubs off the bottom of the base. Then remove any remaining dark green leaves. Using a melon baller, remove the hairy choke from the base of the artichoke. Place the prepared artichoke heart in a bowl of cold water that has had the juice of 1 lemon mixed in to prevent browning.

Tagine of Root Vegetables

A tagine is a traditional dish from the north of Africa. A kind of stew, it is cooked in an earthenware pot with a conical lid, a tagine, which also serves as the serving bowl. In Asia, a similar pot and style of cooking, known as nabe, is a tradition. This stew, combining root and ground vegetables with fragrant spices, creates a wonderful energy in us. When vegetables are stewed, their energies join together to create a unified force in the body, a gathering of strength. Add to that the sparkling energy of spices and you create a dish that gathers your forces, but puts spring in your step. ■ MAKES 5 TO 6 SERVINGS

2 teaspoons extra-virgin olive oil

1 red onion, halved, each half cut into 4 wedges

2 to 3 carrots, 1-inch rolled irregular chunk pieces

½ teaspoon ground coriander

½ teaspoon ground cumin

1 teaspoon hot chile paste

1 cup 1-inch butternut squash cubes

6 to 8 Brussels sprouts, bottoms trimmed, left whole

6 to 8 button mushrooms, stems trimmed, brushed free of dirt, left whole

Soy sauce

Spring or filtered water

1 to 2 teaspoons kuzu, dissolved in 1 tablespoon cold water

Small handful fresh cilantro, minced, for garnish

Heat the oil in a clay tagine or nabe pot over medium heat. Add the onion and sauté until limp, about 1 minute. Add the carrots, coriander, and cumin and stir well. Stir in the chile paste and cook over low heat about 5 minutes, stirring occasionally. Add the squash, Brussels sprouts, and mushrooms. Add a dash of soy sauce and enough water to make ½ inch liquid in the bottom of the pot. Cover and bring to a boil over medium heat. Reduce heat to low and simmer until the squash is quite soft, about 25 minutes. Season lightly with soy sauce and simmer 3 to 4 minutes more. Gently stir in dissolved kuzu, taking care not to break the vegetables too much. Cook, stirring gently, until a thin glaze forms over the vegetables. Serve immediately, garnished with cilantro.

Baked Squash with Pan-Roasted Vegetables

Sweet acorn squash is richly seasoned and baked and then stuffed with pan-roasted root veggies that are infused with Asian flavors. The combination is splendid, as you bring together the complementary tastes and energies of the various ingredients. This dish leaves you feeling satisfied and energized and looking vital and youthful, as the middle organs relax and keep the energy in the body moving smoothly. ▪ MAKES 4 MAIN-COURSE SERVINGS

2 medium acorn squash, halved lengthwise, seeded

Light sesame oil

2 pinches sea salt

About 2 tablespoons barley malt

3 tablespoons extra-virgin olive oil

1 onion, cut into large dice

2 medium turnips, halved lengthwise, cut into 1-inch cubes

2 medium rutabagas, halved lengthwise, cut into 1-inch cubes

2 parsnips, cut into 1-inch rolled irregular chunk pieces

1-inch piece fresh ginger, grated, juice extracted (see Note, page 201)

Soy sauce

1 to 2 tablespoons mirin

Preheat oven to 400F (205C). Lightly oil a baking sheet.

Rub the squash halves lightly with sesame oil, then salt and barley malt (use your fingers; it makes the work easier). Place the squash, cut side down, on the baking sheet and bake, uncovered, until tender and browned, about 40 minutes.

Heat the olive oil in an ovenproof cast-iron skillet. Add the onion and sauté for 1 minute. Add the remaining vegetables and cook over medium heat, 5 to 7 minutes, stirring frequently to prevent scorching. Add the ginger juice, soy sauce to taste, and mirin. Stir well and cook for 1 to 2 minutes. Transfer skillet to oven and roast vegetables, uncovered, 25 to 30 minutes, or until tender and browned, stirring occasionally to ensure even browning. (You can cook the pan-roasted vegetables at the same time as the squash, on different racks.)

To serve, place the squash halves, cut side up, on a serving platter and mound roasted vegetables in each cavity, filling abundantly. Serve hot or warm.

Winter Squash and Carrot Puree

The combination of sweet ground vegetables and strong root vegetables is one of the most wonderful beauty treatments I can imagine. These splendid energies

come together to create a calm endurance that prevents stress from taking its toll on our body and how it functions, and ultimately, how we look as we go through life. A body that is free of tight muscles and stiff joints is a body that maintains a youthful posture and a relaxed, confident stride. Organ systems that function smoothly, free of constriction and stagnation, result in a face with clear elastic skin and strong, shiny hair. ■ MAKES 5 TO 6 SERVINGS

2 medium butternut squash, peeled, seeded, cut into 1-inch cubes

8 to 10 carrots, cut into 1-inch rolled, irregular pieces

2 tablespoons brown rice syrup

¼ cup light olive oil

¼ cup plain soy milk

¼ teaspoon ground cinnamon

Sea salt

Cinnamon sticks, for garnish

Place the squash and carrots in a heavy saucepan. Add the rice syrup and oil and bring to a boil, uncovered, over medium heat. Add the soy milk, ground cinnamon, and 2 pinches of salt, cover, and return to the boil. Reduce heat to low and simmer until vegetables are quite soft, about 25 minutes.

Using a food mill, puree the vegetables and remaining liquid in batches to form a silken puree. Transfer to a serving bowl and serve warm, garnished with whole cinnamon sticks.

Sweet Onion Baklava

Is dry skin a problem? Then try this recipe. Not only is it one of the most delicious dishes you will ever taste, it's made from onions, which are moisture-rich and luxurious. The best part is that their strong, rooted nature draws that moisture deep into the body to nourish the skin, keeping it soft and supple, while their peppery, sweet flavor ensures that we will have energy to burn.

■ MAKES 24 SERVINGS

ONION FILLING

About 3 tablespoons extra-virgin olive oil

8 to 10 yellow onions, cut into thin half-moon slices

Sea salt

2 tablespoons brown rice syrup

1-inch piece fresh ginger, grated, juice extracted (see Note, page 201)

1 tablespoon kuzu, dissolved in 3 tablespoons cold water

PASTRY

2 cups blanched almonds

½ teaspoon ground cinnamon (optional)

15 sheets phyllo dough, thawed in the refrigerator, laid flat on a dry surface
and covered with a kitchen towel

About ½ cup extra-virgin olive oil

To make the filling: Heat the olive oil in a deep skillet over medium heat. Add the onions and sauté with a generous sprinkle of salt until limp, about 5 minutes. Reduce heat to medium-low and cook onions, covered, for 15 minutes, stirring occasionally to prevent scorching. Add the rice syrup and ginger juice and cook, uncovered, until the mixture thickens slightly, about 10 minutes. Stir in the dissolved kuzu and cook, stirring, until the mixture thickens and turns clear, about 3 minutes more. Set aside to cool.

To make the pastry: Preheat oven to 350F (175C). Lightly oil the bottom and sides of a 13 × 9-inch baking pan. Place blanched almonds in a food processor and grind into a fine meal. Add cinnamon, if using, and pulse just to combine.

Fold one sheet of phyllo in half crosswise and fit into prepared pan. Brush lightly with oil. Repeat folding and layering with 4 more sheets of phyllo, creating a multilayered base. Sprinkle evenly with ½ cup of the ground almonds. Spread half the onion filling over almonds and sprinkle with another ½ cup of the ground almonds.

Fold, layer, and oil 5 more phyllo sheets over filling. Sprinkle with ½ cup of the ground almonds and top with remaining onion filling. Sprinkle with ¼ cup almond mixture.

Fold, layer, and oil the remaining 5 sheets of phyllo over the second layer of filling, except in this layer, sprinkle a little of the remaining almond mixture between each folded sheet. Brush the top of the baklava lightly with oil. With a sharp knife, score the top sheets (diamond shapes are most common for this dish, but any shape is okay) to mark 24 servings. Bake on the center oven rack about 50 minutes, or until the phyllo is golden brown and crispy. Remove from oven and cool in the pan on a wire cooling rack. Cut into marked servings and serve warm.

TIPS When you buy phyllo, it usually is in the freezer section. Before use, simply place the package in the refrigerator for about 6 hours to thaw. If you try to thaw frozen phyllo at room temperature, it will soften unevenly, resulting in unusable pastry.

You may purchase blanched almonds in specialty stores or you may blanch almonds by boiling them for 5 minutes, cooling to room temperature, and slipping the brown, papery skins off the nuts.

Lemon-Glazed Brussels Sprouts, Shallots, and Radishes

Vegetables that grow close to the ground have the ability to relax any tension in our middle organs—the spleen, pancreas, and stomach—resulting in regulated blood sugar levels and a calm, centered attitude. When our bodies are relaxed and blood sugars normalized, our skin takes on a healthy glow, free of red splotches and blemishes. ■ MAKES 5 TO 6 SERVINGS

10 to 12 Brussels sprouts, trimmed, bottoms scored with an X, left whole

½ cup brown rice syrup

Grated zest of 1 lemon, plus extra for garnish

2 onions, halved, each half cut into 4 wedges

8 to 10 red radishes, cleaned, trimmed, left whole

Soy sauce

1 cup spring or filtered water

Pinch of ground cardamom

Juice of ½ lemon

Bring a pot of water to a boil. Add the Brussels sprouts and boil for 3 minutes to begin to tenderize them. Drain and set aside.

In a deep skillet, combine the rice syrup and lemon zest. Cook over low heat for about 5 minutes. Stir in the onions and radishes, season lightly with soy sauce, and add the water and cardamom. Bring to a boil over medium heat, reduce heat to low, and simmer, uncovered, until the vegetables are soft, about 15 minutes. Stir in the Brussels sprouts and cook until they are soft and the liquid has reduced to a thick syrup, about 10 minutes more. Turn off heat and gently stir in the lemon juice. Serve warm, garnished with lemon zest.

TIP When cooking with citrus juice, remember that you want a delicate tart flavor, so do not overcook it. Either add it at the end of cooking (so it simmers no more than 1 minute), or stir in after cooking is complete. This way, the juice does not become bitter and the delicate tartness is preserved.

Lemony Cucumber Salad

Water retention is one of women's more common complaints. It can give us puffy eyes and cheeks, swollen fingers and feet, and make us feel ever so unattractive. Did you know that water retention is caused by excess intake of simple sugars, not just salt as is commonly believed?

The good news is that some diet adjustments and lightly tart astringent salads like this one can bring our bodies back into balance. The sour flavors will help stagnant energy move and the delicate diuretic nature of the cucumber will help to balance our liquids, with the carrot helping the body to do its work most effectively. ▪ MAKES 4 TO 5 SERVINGS

2 to 3 cucumbers

6 scallions, thinly sliced on the diagonal

1 red bell pepper, roasted over an open flame, peeled, seeded, thinly sliced
    into strips (see Note, page 178)

1 carrot, cut into fine matchstick pieces, blanched for 30 seconds, drained

2 tablespoons minced flat-leaf parsley

LEMONY DRESSING

½ cup plain soy milk

Sea salt

Grated zest of 1 lemon

½ teaspoon kuzu, dissolved in 1 teaspoon cold water

Juice of 1 lemon

If you are using organic cucumbers, leave the peel on. However, if you are using nonorganic cucumbers, remove the waxed peel. Cut off both tips of the cucumber and rub it in a circular motion crosswise over the tip. You will notice a thick, white paste draw from the vegetable. This paste is the cause of indigestion and so is best if removed. Halve the cucumbers lengthwise and slice on the diagonal into very thin half-moon slices. Combine the cucumbers with remaining vegetables and parsley, cover, and chill.

To make the dressing: Combine the soy milk, a generous pinch of salt, and lemon zest in a saucepan. Warm through over low heat. Stir in the dissolved kuzu and cook, stirring, until the mixture thickens, about 3 minutes. Whisk in the lemon juice and spoon over chilled salad. Serve immediately to get the full benefit of the warm dressing atop the chilled vegetables.

Shiitake and Scallion Pâté

No one feasting on this pâté at your dinner party will know that you are truly the perfect host. Not only is the food delicious, but you are recharging their kidneys with this starter dish whose rich taste belies its benefits. With the shiitake mushrooms to relax any stagnant energy and tight muscles and the scallion to make your energy sparkle, this delicious pâté will do more than start your meal, it will relax your guests, and help them get rid of their aching lower backs.

■ MAKES 4 TO 5 SERVINGS

About 2 teaspoons extra-virgin olive oil

2 to 3 shallots, finely minced

1-inch piece fresh ginger, grated, juice extracted (see Note, page 201)

Pinch of sea salt

8 to 10 dried shiitake mushrooms, soaked until soft, finely minced

8 to 10 button mushrooms, brushed free of dirt, finely minced

2 teaspoons soy sauce

1 tablespoon brown rice vinegar

1 teaspoon umeboshi vinegar or vinegar

2 teaspoons mirin

2 teaspoons brown rice syrup

4 ounces firm tofu

1 bunch scallions, trimmed, thinly sliced

1 bunch watercress, rinsed, lightly blanched, and thinly sliced

Toast points or vegetable sticks, to serve

Heat 1 to 2 teaspoons oil in a skillet over medium heat. Add the shallots, ginger juice, and salt and sauté until limp, about 1 minute. Add the shiitake mushrooms and sauté 1 minute. Stir in the button mushrooms and sauté until the mushrooms release their juices and begin to reabsorb them, about 5 minutes. Transfer the mushroom mixture to a shallow baking dish.

Mix together the soy sauce, vinegars, mirin, and rice syrup and pour over cooked mushrooms. Set aside to marinate for 15 minutes.

Drain the mushroom mixture and transfer it to a food processor. Add the tofu and scallions and puree until smooth and thick.

To serve, press the pâté into a lightly oiled bowl, smoothing the pâté top until flat. Arrange the watercress on a plate and invert bowl with pâté on the center. Serve with toast points or vegetable sticks.

Thai Cabbage Slaw

The combinations of energies in this dish will make you smile. Spicy flavors will vitalize you by increasing circulation and energy flow through the body; cucumbers jump in to dampen down the flames a bit, while relaxing your body. This is all set against the backdrop of the splendidly calming green cabbage, whose delicate sweetness and centered nature create a dish that will have you looking alert and clear-eyed. ▪ MAKES 4 TO 5 SERVINGS

½ head green cabbage, finely shredded

1 carrot, cut into fine matchstick pieces

1 cucumber, cut into fine matchstick pieces

3 to 4 scallions, cut into 1-inch pieces

½ cup loosely packed fresh basil leaves, shredded

THAI-SPICED DRESSING

3 tablespoons toasted sesame oil

¼ cup sesame tahini

2 tablespoons brown rice vinegar

1 teaspoon soy sauce

2 teaspoons Thai curry paste

Spring or filtered water

Basil sprigs, to garnish

Bring a pot of water to a boil and lightly blanch the cabbage, about 1 minute. Remove with a slotted spoon, drain well, and transfer to a mixing bowl. Blanch the carrot for 30 seconds, drain, and add to cabbage. Mix in the cucumber, scallions, and basil. Toss gently to combine.

To make the dressing: Whisk all ingredients, except water and basil, in a small bowl until smooth. Slowly add enough water to achieve the consistency you desire. A thicker dressing will coat the vegetables more evenly than a thin one. Warm dressing over low heat for 5 minutes.

Stir dressing into vegetable mixture to combine. Set aside for 30 minutes before serving to develop the flavors. Stir gently before serving. Serve warm or chilled, garnished with basil sprigs.

Ginger-Glazed Broccoli

There's nothing quite like ginger (other than running a marathon) for stimulating circulation, which leaves us looking just great. In this dish, ginger teams up with broccoli, one of our best sources for calcium, folic acid, and vitamin C, and as a result creates exquisite hair and strong nails. When we eat broccoli, we merge our energy, with it, allowing us to tap into the vegetable's vitality.

■ MAKES 4 TO 5 SERVINGS

2 to 3 stalks broccoli, stems trimmed, peeled, thinly sliced, cut into small florets

¼ cup light sesame oil

3 tablespoons finely minced fresh ginger

1 teaspoon powdered ginger

3 tablespoons brown rice syrup

½ teaspoon soy sauce

Slivered lemon zest, to garnish

Bring a pot of water to a boil. Add the broccoli stems and cook until crisp-tender, about 1 minute. Remove with a slotted spoon, drain, and set aside. Cook the broccoli florets until bright green and crisp-tender, about 2 minutes. Drain and mix with stems.

In a skillet, cook the oil, fresh ginger, powdered ginger, rice syrup, and soy sauce over medium-low heat until slightly thickened, about 5 minutes. Add the broccoli to the hot syrup and stir to coat. Transfer to a serving platter, drizzling any remaining syrup over top. Serve garnished with lemon zest.

Asian Wild Green Salad

Wild greens' bitter flavor and unbridled vitality (hence the word wild as their description) give us energy to burn as well as nourishing and helping to cleanse the liver. The benefits to your looks are no creases between the brows, clear whites of the eyes, and even skin tone. ■ MAKES 2 TO 3 SERVINGS

½ cup slivered almonds

Light olive oil, for frying

4 ounces extra-firm tofu, cut into small cubes

About 2 teaspoons extra-virgin oil

1 tablespoon finely minced fresh ginger

½ teaspoon chile powder

1 small leek, split lengthwise, rinsed, thinly sliced

Soy sauce

Mirin

1 red bell pepper, roasted over an open flame, peeled, seeded, sliced into thin
    strips (see Note, page 178)

2 to 3 dried shiitake mushrooms, soaked until soft, drained, thinly sliced

¼ cup shredded fresh basil

2 to 3 tablespoons shredded fresh mint (optional)

1 bunch dandelion greens, arugula, broccoli rabe, or watercress, rinsed well,
    thinly sliced

1 cup mung bean sprouts

Juice of 1 lime

Lime wedges, for garnish

Preheat oven to 350F (175C). Arrange the almonds on a baking sheet
and bake about 5 minutes, or until lightly browned. Set aside to cool.

In a medium saucepan, heat about 1 inch of olive oil over medium
heat. Make sure the oil is hot enough by submerging the handle of a
wooden spoon in the oil. If bubbles gather around the tips, the oil is
ready. Increase the heat to high, add the tofu, and fry until golden,
turning cubes to brown evenly. Drain on paper towels and set aside.

Heat the extra-virgin olive oil in a wok over medium heat. Add the
ginger, chile powder, and leek and sauté for about 1 minute. Sprinkle
lightly with soy sauce and mirin, add the bell pepper, and stir well. Add
the shiitake mushrooms, basil, and mint if using, sprinkle lightly with
soy sauce, and stir-fry for about 1 minute. Stir in the greens and mung
bean sprouts, season lightly with soy sauce, and stir-fry until the greens
are just limp, 3 to 4 minutes.

Just before serving, squeeze the lime juice over the greens mixture, add the fried tofu and almonds, and toss to combine. Serve with lime wedges on the side.

Veggie and Bread Salad with Corn

This rustic salad is truly delicious, and its balance is remarkable. Combining sharp and sweet flavors with a rich dressing serves us in many ways. Sharp taste will help tone the liver, creating clear eyes and even coloring. Sweet taste will relax the middle organs, leaving our faces line-free, and the rich dressing will moisturize our skin from the inside out. The astringent quality of the greens ensures good digestion. ■ MAKES 5 TO 6 SERVINGS

1 cup fresh or frozen corn kernels

1 carrot, cut into very thin oblong pieces

1 red onion, cut into thin half-moon slices

1 small bunch broccoli rabe, rinsed well, left whole

5 to 6 slices whole-grain sourdough bread, crusts removed, cut into 1-inch cubes

6 to 8 red radishes, thinly sliced

1 to 2 cucumbers, thinly sliced on the diagonal

12 to 15 oil-cured black olives, pitted, finely chopped

DRESSING

½ cup extra-virgin olive oil

2 to 3 tablespoons balsamic vinegar

2 teaspoons umeboshi vinegar or 2 teaspoons fresh lemon juice and ½ teaspoon sea salt

1 teaspoon sea salt

5 to 6 fresh basil leaves, finely minced

Bring a pot of water to a boil. Blanch the corn for about 30 seconds, remove with a slotted spoon, drain, and place in a mixing bowl. Blanch the carrot for about 1 minute, remove with a slotted spoon, drain, and add to the corn. Blanch the red onion for about 30 seconds, remove with a slotted spoon, drain, and add to the corn and carrot. Blanch the broccoli rabe for about 1 minute, drain, and cut into bite-size pieces. Mix the broccoli rabe, bread cubes, radishes, cucumbers, and olives into the corn mixture.

To make the dressing: Whisk the ingredients together in a small bowl until smooth. Adjust flavor to your taste. Stir dressing gently into vegetable and bread mixture and set aside to marinate for at least 1 hour before serving. The longer the salad can marinate, the better the flavors will develop. Stir occasionally as the salad marinates.

Watercress and Fried Mushroom Salad

There's nothing like the clean, peppery taste of watercress to make you look your best. A great liver tonic, watercress can aid the body in cleansing itself of toxins, giving us great-looking skin and clear, bright eyes, with eye whites that are white. Adding sautéed mushroom to the mix moisturizes the skin and hair and cleanses fat deposits from the veins and arteries, making our skin look fresh and alive.

■ MAKES 4 SERVINGS

12 dried shiitake mushrooms, soaked until soft

1 cup plain soy milk

Sea salt

Yellow cornmeal, for dredging

1 red onion, cut into ¼-inch-thick rings

2 bunches watercress, rinsed well, left whole

Light olive oil, for frying

SESAME DRESSING

3 tablespoons sesame tahini

½ teaspoon umeboshi vinegar

½ teaspoon soy sauce

Juice of 1 lemon

1 teaspoon fresh ginger juice (see Note, page 201)

1 teaspoon brown rice syrup

Spring or filtered water

Drain the mushrooms, reserve the soaking liquid, and discard the stems. Place the mushrooms in a saucepan with the soy milk and a generous pinch of salt. Bring to a boil, uncovered, over medium heat. Reduce heat to low and simmer until mushrooms are tender, about 15 minutes. Drain the mushrooms and dredge in cornmeal to coat. Set aside.

Bring a pot of water to a boil. Blanch the onion for about 30 seconds, remove with a slotted spoon, drain, and lay on a platter. Blanch the watercress about 30 seconds, drain, and slice into bite-size pieces. Set aside to cool.

Heat about 1 inch of olive oil in a deep pot over medium heat. While the oil heats, make the dressing: Whisk the ingredients together in a small bowl until smooth, slowly adding water until you achieve the desired consistency. Set aside.

When the oil is hot, increase the heat to high and quickly fry the mushrooms until crispy golden brown. Drain on paper towels.

To serve, arrange watercress and onion on individual salad plates. Top each salad with 3 mushrooms. Drizzle with dressing and serve immediately.

Bruschetta with Sautéed Bitter Greens

This is a great way to enjoy greens, especially if they are relatively new to your repertoire of foods. The sautéing adds a rich, comforting energy and vitality and the toasted bread adds a crunchy texture that is irresistible. This simple side dish is your ticket to clear, bright eyes, a line-free brow, and an even complexion. The bitter taste and astringent quality of the greens will relax the liver, enhancing its ability to rid the body of accumulated toxins. The olive oil will moisturize the skin. ▪ MAKES 4 SERVINGS

> 8 slices whole-grain sourdough baguette
> About 2 tablespoons extra-virgin olive oil
> Sea salt
> ½ dried chile pepper, seeded and diced
> 1 bunch broccoli rabe, rinsed well, thinly sliced

Preheat the oven to 350F (175C). Line a baking sheet with parchment paper.

Arrange the bread slices on the baking sheet. Brush lightly with some of the oil and sprinkle lightly with salt. Bake about 15 minutes, or until crisp and golden.

While the bread toasts, heat 1 tablespoon oil in a deep skillet and add the chile pepper and sauté until fragrant. Stir in the broccoli rabe, season lightly with salt, and sauté over medium-high heat until broccoli rabe is deep green and just tender, about 5 minutes.

To serve, arrange toasts on a platter and mound each with sautéed broccoli rabe. Serve hot.

Hearty Greens with Spiced Walnuts

Relaxing tension in the body to look our best, doesn't mean creating couch potatoes. When the body is free of tension, it can use energy efficiently, and you feel vital and strong. This special warm salad is ideal to increase energy with relaxed flexibility. Steaming the greens brings their character into focus. They are our greatest ally for good-looking skin and hair. Add to them sweetly cooked fruit for a line-free face and spiced nuts for vitality (remember, nuts grow entire trees and spices enliven our energy), and you have a dish that will put a spring in your step. ■ MAKES 4 TO 5 SERVINGS

6 tablespoons plus 1 teaspoon brown rice syrup

1 cup plus 2 tablespoons spring or filtered water

Dash soy sauce

½ teaspoon powdered ginger

Pinch ground cinnamon

1 cup walnut pieces

½ cup unsweetened dried cranberries

Pinch sea salt

1 bunch kale, rinsed well, stems trimmed, left whole

Preheat oven to 325F (175C). Line a baking sheet with parchment paper.

In a small saucepan, warm the 6 tablespoons rice syrup, 2 tablespoons water, soy sauce, and spices for 2 minutes. Remove from heat and fold in the walnuts. Spread on the prepared baking sheet and bake about 15 minutes, or until golden brown. Set aside.

Combine the cranberries with the 1 cup water, salt, and the 1 teaspoon rice syrup and simmer over medium-low heat until plump, 10 minutes. Drain and set aside.

In a large pot, bring ½ inch of water to a boil. Place the kale, stem ends down, in pot. Cover and steam until deep green and just tender, about 3 minutes. Drain and slice into bite-size pieces.

To serve, arrange kale on a platter, top with cranberries and nuts, and serve.

Orange-Sesame Asparagus

It doesn't get easier than this delicious dish, and what the dish does for you is even better. Asparagus, the epitome of spring, has the ability to refresh the body by acting as a mild diuretic, so we don't look puffy. It can also direct our energy up and out, so we feel lighter and fresher. The result is a spring in your step, fresh, clear skin, and distinct features. ▪ MAKES 4 TO 5 SERVINGS

1 pound fresh asparagus, ends snapped off

1 teaspoon light sesame oil

2 to 3 shallots, finely minced

1 carrot, finely minced

Soy sauce

1 to 2 teaspoons black sesame seeds, lightly toasted

Juice of 1 orange

Orange slices, for garnish

In a large pot of boiling water, cook the asparagus until bright green and crisp-tender, about 4 minutes. Drain and set aside.

Heat the oil in a sauté pan over medium heat. Add the shallots and sauté 1 minute. Add the carrot, season lightly with soy sauce, and sauté

2 minutes more. Add the sesame seeds and orange juice, stir to combine, and remove from heat.

To serve, lay asparagus spears on a platter and spoon the carrot mixture over the top. Garnish with orange slices and serve.

TIPS Snapping the ends off asparagus spears ensures that the tips break in the natural place. If you cut the ends off the asparagus, you may not remove all of the tough parts, or even worse, too much of the tender stalk. A great way to cook asparagus stalks is in a fish poaching pan. The spears lay flat and maintain their straight shape.

Collard Greens with Caramelized Onions and Pine Nuts

Just when you think you can't face another side dish of steamed greens, give this recipe a try. It's not quite as easy as steaming, but the flavor and energy are so lovely, you won't mind a few more minutes of preparation. Because eating greens is so deeply connected to how well our skin ages, their value is without compare, but we need variety to keep our interest. ■ MAKES 3 TO 4 SERVINGS

>2 teaspoons light sesame oil
>
>1 red onion, cut into thin half-moon slices
>
>Soy sauce
>
>½ cup pine nuts
>
>1 small bunch collard greens, rinsed, stems trimmed

Heat the oil in a deep skillet over medium heat. Add the onion and sauté with a dash of soy sauce until limp and beginning to brown, about 15 minutes, stirring frequently. Add the pine nuts and stir to combine. Spread the onion and pine nuts over the bottom of the skillet. Slice the greens into ½-inch strips just before placing in the skillet. Sprinkle lightly with soy sauce, cover, and reduce heat to medium-low. Cook until greens are bright green and just tender, about 5 minutes. Stir well to combine ingredients and serve.

Endive, Escarole, and Pear Salad

The combination of fresh and cooked vegetables ensures that the body's energy stays strong, but with a light, fresh quality. The bitterness of the greens will relax the liver, creating whites of the eyes free of bloodshot veins as well as minimizing those little wrinkles between the brows. The sweet fruit will relax the middle body so that your face looks stress-free, even though your life may not be.

■ MAKES 4 SERVING

2 Belgian endive, ends trimmed, quartered lengthwise

Extra-virgin olive oil

Soy sauce

Mirin

1 head escarole, rinsed very well, torn into small pieces

2 pears, halved, cored, thinly sliced, tossed in lemon juice to prevent discoloration

LEMON-SOY VINAIGRETTE

3 tablespoons brown rice vinegar

2 tablespoons extra virgin olive oil

1 tablespoon soy sauce

Juice of 1 lemon

2 teaspoons brown rice syrup

½ cup pecans, lightly toasted, for garnish

Preheat oven to 375F (190C). Arrange endive quarters in a shallow baking dish and lightly drizzle with olive oil, soy sauce, and mirin. Bake, uncovered, 20 to 30 minutes, or until tender and edges are just browned.

While the endive bakes, arrange the escarole on a platter. Chill pear slices until ready to serve.

Make the vinaigrette: Whisk the ingredients together in a small bowl to combine. Adjust flavor to your taste. Set aside.

To serve, arrange the chilled pear slices on top of the escarole, top with the endive spears, sprinkle with the pecans, and drizzle generously with dressing. Serve immediately.

TIP Chilling the pears adds a wonderful crispness to them, as well as creating the delightful combination of cold and hot ingredients to stimulate your appetite.

Summer Hiziki Salad

Hiziki is a gold mine of nutrition, with concentrated amounts of calcium, vitamin D, and protein all coming together to create deep strength and vitality. This dish helps to create strong, efficient intestines, which gives us strong, lustrous hair with nary a split end. You heard right, a bit of hiziki in your diet and it's bye-bye ragged ends. ▪ MAKES ABOUT 4 SERVINGS

½ cup dried hiziki, soaked until soft, diced

Soy sauce

Mirin

1 small yellow squash, cut into fine matchstick pieces

1 carrot, cut into fine matchstick pieces

1 bunch watercress, rinsed well, left whole

1 cucumber

DRESSING

3 tablespoons sesame tahini

Juice of 1 lemon

3 to 4 scallions, finely minced

1 teaspoon brown rice syrup

Spring or filtered water

Place the hiziki in a saucepan with enough water to just cover. Season lightly with soy sauce and mirin and bring to a boil, uncovered. Reduce heat to low, cover, and cook until hiziki is tender, about 25 minutes. Remove cover, increase heat to medium, and cook away any remaining liquid.

Bring a pot of water to a boil and blanch the yellow squash until crisp-tender, about 1 minute. Remove with a slotted spoon, drain, and transfer to a mixing bowl. Blanch the carrot until crisp-tender, about 1 minute, remove with a slotted spoon, drain, and mix in with squash. Finally, blanch the watercress, drain, and cut into bite-size pieces. Mix in with the carrot and squash. Thinly slice the cucumber on the diagonal, place in a covered bowl, and chill completely.

To make the dressing: Whisk all ingredients, except water, together in a small bowl. Slowly whisk in enough water to achieve the desired consistency.

To serve, arrange chilled cucumber slices around the rim of a platter. Make a wide mound of blanched vegetables in the center, with a small mound of hiziki on top. Drizzle generously with dressing and serve.

Nori Rolls with Greens and Portobellos

When you think of nori, you think of sushi rice and veggies wrapped in this richly flavored sea plant. But nori rolls can constitute many kinds of side dishes, so use your imagination. High in calcium, vitamin D, and some B vitamins, nori is a valuable ingredient in making your skin, hair, and nails their very best.

■ MAKES 4 TO 5 SERVINGS

> 3 portobello mushrooms
> Light sesame oil
> Soy sauce
> Mirin
> 12 to 16 (⅛-inch-thick) carrot spears
> 1 small bunch collard greens (12 to 16 leaves), stems trimmed, left whole
> 3 to 4 sheets toasted nori
> Soy dipping sauce (optional)

Preheat oven to 375F (175C). Arrange the mushrooms in a shallow baking dish and drizzle lightly with oil, soy sauce, and mirin. Bake, uncovered, about 25 minutes, or until tender. Remove from oven, allow to cool, and cut into thin slices.

Bring a pot of water to a boil and cook carrot spears until tender, about 2 minutes. Remove with a slotted spoon, drain, and set aside. Boil collard greens until just tender, about 2 minutes. Drain and lay flat on a platter.

To assemble the rolls, lay a sheet of nori, shiny side down, against a bamboo sushi mat or kitchen towel. Lay 2 to 3 collard leaves lengthwise on the nori. Lay carrot spears and portobello slices, the length of the nori roll, on the side of the greens closest to you. Using the mat as a guide, firmly roll the nori and greens around the mushrooms and carrots, forming a firm cylinder. Repeat with remaining ingredients.

To serve, slice each nori roll into 8 equal pieces and arrange, cut side up, on a platter. Serve with a soy dipping sauce, if desired.

Pan-Fried Arame with Spring Vegetables

Arame has the ability to draw toxins and excess fluids from the body, so much so, that we can even use its soaking water in our bath to relieve water retention. In our diet, arame helps us achieve the same kind of internal moisture balance. Seems like a great trade-off, a bit of seaweed to avoid bloating.

■ MAKES 4 TO 5 SERVINGS

½ cup dried arame

4 to 5 teaspoons light sesame oil

Soy sauce

½ leek, split lengthwise, rinsed well, thinly sliced

1 carrot, cut into fine matchstick pieces

¼ head red cabbage, finely shredded

2 cups green beans, tips trimmed, left whole

3 to 4 leaves kale, rinsed, left whole

Umeboshi vinegar or lemon juice

Brown rice vinegar

Rinse arame several times and set aside in a bowl to soften; soaking is not needed. Cut into small pieces.

Heat 2 teaspoons of the oil in a small skillet over medium heat. Add the arame and sauté with a generous dash of soy sauce for 1 minute. Reduce heat to medium-low and cook, stirring occasionally, about 15 minutes. If the arame begins to stick to the pan, add a little water, but not too much or you will flatten the flavor.

While the arame cooks, heat the remaining oil in a wok over medium heat. Add the leek and sauté with a dash of soy sauce for 1 minute. Add the carrot, cabbage, and a dash of soy sauce and sauté 1 to 2 minutes. Stir in the green beans and a dash of soy sauce and sauté for 1 minute. Slice and stir in the kale, season to taste with soy sauce, cover the wok, and cook over medium heat until kale is a rich green and tender, about 3 minutes. Stir the arame into kale mixture, sprinkle with vinegars to taste, toss to combine, and serve.

Cucumber-Wakame Salsa

Just a touch of sea vegetables goes a long way, so be creative. Their strong flavors and concentrated nutrients make them perfect as relishes, small side dishes, or, as in this case, salsa. With the ability to maintain strong blood, particularly red blood cells, these exotic veggies from the sea help to create lustrous hair, strong nails, and a flawless complexion. ■ MAKES 5 TO 6 SERVINGS

½ cup dried wakame, soaked until soft, finely minced

2 cucumbers, finely diced

4 to 5 red radishes, finely diced

2 to 3 scallions, finely minced

2 teaspoons umeboshi vinegar

2 teaspoons brown rice vinegar

Juice of 1 lime

1 teaspoon soy sauce

1 teaspoon mirin

2 to 3 cups mesclun greens, rinsed well

Combine the wakame, cucumbers, radishes, and scallions in a mixing bowl. Whisk together the vinegars, lime juice, soy sauce, and mirin in a small bowl. Adjust seasoning to your taste. Stir dressing into vegetable mixture and toss to combine. Set aside to marinate for at least 1 hour before serving to allow flavors to develop. Serve at room temperature or chilled.

Arrange greens on a plate and spoon salsa over the top.

Beans for Beauty

We've been conditioned to worry about protein. I think it all began back in the '70s, when large numbers of young Americans began to experiment with vegetarianism, myself included. Many conventional nutritionists began issuing warnings on the dangers of protein deficiency. Their theory was that health couldn't be maintained on a diet that excluded animal protein. The general feeling seemed to be that unless a vegetarian diet was heavily supplemented, anyone eating a plant-based diet was on the fast track to malnutrition. They're not entirely wrong. Without the proper balance of nutrients, vegetarians, particularly vegans, can find it difficult to get enough of certain nutrients, like vitamin B-12. Vegans (myself included) may need to seriously consider the possibility of supplements, particularly with the quality of our food supply being compromised more every year with pollution, genetic modification, and pesticide use.

History shows us the cultural importance of protein. In many societies, including our own, the ability to serve animal flesh at the table signified affluence and security. It was a sign of the prosperity of an entire society. Even during our own Depression era, we were promised "a chicken in every pot" as an illustration that there was a light at the end of the tunnel during those dark economic times. In other cultures, the hunter was revered above all men for his ability to feed the tribe. And so with our attitudes being shaped by so many factors, cultural and historical, we feel especially attached to protein and consider it essential to our survival.

Protein is special in many ways. It is the only nutrient that contains nitrogen. Protein is composed of complex molecules and gives organisms their biological character, their identity, if you will. However, in general nutrition terms, our bodies need protein, carbohydrates, and fats. To eliminate or excessively consume one over the other will create an imbalance in the body that impedes us on our quest to look and feel great.

So what's the deal with protein? How much do we need and where should we look for it? The good news is that vegetable protein is not inferior to animal protein, a belief based on the fact that vegetable proteins are not "complete," because some of them are missing some of the essential amino acids, the building blocks that the body can't make. What everyone is forgetting is that the body will glean the missing essential amino acids (and vitamin B-12) from the vast number of bacteria that reside in the lower intestinal tract, as well as from the cells that slough off the lining of the digestive tract on a daily basis. In fact, choosing to eat vegetable protein can actually make you healthier. Studies show that people eating a plant-based diet live better and longer, maintaining a youthful appearance far longer than people eating more flesh.

In addition, human protein needs are lower than we have been conditioned to think they are. Despite what we have been told, especially recently with many high-protein diets being the rage, even athletes and people engaging in heavy physical labor do not need to consume excessive amounts of protein. In this age of protein "experts" (and it seems there is a new one added to the list daily), we know less about protein than we know about carbohydrates or fat. In particular, we seem to understand very little about individual needs. We can't seem to explain why some people need more—or less—protein than others to operate well in life. There are those who thrive on great quantities of protein and find their energy sorely lacking if they don't get enough. And then there are those who find that even one excessive serving of protein in a meal leaves them feeling lethargic and heavy. So the consumption of protein is quite personal and how much we eat depends largely on how we feel when we eat it. It comes down to understanding proteins and how they work in the body. Then you can determine protein needs that are appropriate for you. You become the expert on you.

In whole-foods cooking, the general rule of thumb is that people operate optimally when their diet consists of 50 percent of the calories from complex carbohydrates, about 30 percent from fats, and about 20 percent from protein. Why? Protein consumed in excess of what our bodies need to grow becomes fuel for the body to burn. The problem is that protein is an inefficient fuel compared to carbohydrate-fueled energy. Protein molecules are quite complex, so the ratio of energy gained versus energy burned in metabolism is out of kilter. It requires more energy to metabolize and utilize energy from protein, much more than is required to metabolize the nutrients from carbohydrates and fat. All this means is that fuel from protein makes the body work harder than fuel burned from carbohydrates and fat. It does explain why people initially lose weight and feel energized on a high-protein diet. It also explains why people who consume more protein age differently than those who eat less. The harder the body works to digest, the more tired the body grows; the quicker the skin wrinkles and ages.

The metabolic combustion of protein by the body yields ammonia as waste. The body protects itself from this strong toxin by converting it to urea, a less poisonous substance, a job that is the responsibility of the liver. Then the kidneys get involved, since they have the job of removing urea from the bloodstream and excreting it in our urine. Therefore, excessive consumption of protein overworks the liver and the kidneys and exposes our sensitive internal environment to toxic waste. And while the liver and kidneys are doing their job when they aid the body in eliminating toxins, the overtaxing of these organs deserves our attention, not only in terms of how we look; the impact there is obvious in fine lines between the brows, puffy dark bags under our eyes, and a washed-out, pallid complexion. Dietary protein is a factor in both liver and kidney disease, with doctors carefully monitoring a patient's protein consumption to aid these organs in their struggle with such illness.

Most of us think that eating lots of protein helps to build strong bones, since we associate protein with strength. Protein has the job of building muscle, but when consumed in quantities greater than what our bodies need, it can actually be detrimental to our bones. When the body produces excessive amounts of urea, it requires an increase in water loss in the urine to flush the urea from the system. This strong diuretic effect (another reason for weight loss on a high-protein diet) results in the loss of minerals, especially calcium.

Now as much as I would love to see the whole world live on plant foods, with no animals losing their lives for our feasting, I'm also a realist. We are a culture that has lived on animal flesh for many years and the thought of eliminating that food source appalls many people. I know that some people require the strength they can get from small amounts of animal protein. But I believe that we are suffering, as a species, from our excessive consumption of animal flesh and that our health is suffering as a consequence. If we made other protein choices, we would see an incredible shift in the health of humanity and the planet. We might actually be kinder and gentler, not just use it as the catchphrase for a dream.

RECOMMENDED PROTEIN SOURCES

Plant protein is the best source of protein overall, with small amounts of animal food, if needed, for your personal well-being. Should that be the case for you, the best sources of animal protein and its accompanying strength is fish. On top of that, wild, natural fish, versus farm-raised fish, is your best choice, if you can get it. Farm-raising fish is not only inhumane, but the fish are fed in ways that are less than natural. My personal favorites, for my husband, who eats fish, are wild Alaskan salmon or anything that he might catch himself.

BEST SOURCES OF PLANT PROTEIN

While protein exists in all plants, except fruit, it is especially abundant in beans, bean products, and seeds.

There is much good news about beans and bean products. Rich in protein, they also contain complex carbohydrates (the low glycemic index type). They also contain fat, fiber, folic acid, and phytochemicals. The only bad news with beans is that they require longer cooking to be easily digested and may carry in them pesticide residues in concentrated amounts, unless you are using certified organic beans, which I highly recommend. Taking protein from plants rather than animals has other advantages as well. Certainly less expensive than animal flesh, plant proteins are also less perishable. Lower in saturated fatty acids than animal flesh, the fat in beans is better for our health. The higher fiber and carbohydrate content in plant protein makes them less concentrated than animal protein, so they are easier to digest and are lighter, allowing you to eat a larger volume of them, without overloading the system with protein.

As you might guess from my long essays on whole ingredients, I'm not a big fan of protein powders, supplements, and other forms of processed plant proteins, as they are devoid of vital life-giving energy.

WHAT TO BUY

Before you rush off to the natural-foods store and load up on all sorts of dried beans, take a breath and read on. You don't want to become overwhelmed by introducing too many variables into the picture. Start with a few types of dried beans, a block of tofu, and a package of tempeh. Green lentils, red adzuki beans, and chickpeas are great for starting to cook with beans. All of them are easy to prepare, with shorter cooking times, and they are sweetly flavored, so you'll like them. They are nourishing to the skin and hair, since they are low in fat and very relaxing to the middle organs of the body, making them beneficial to digestion.

Tofu and tempeh fall under the magical soy category and are important additions to your repertoire of beans. Soybeans and their products have long been prized by generations of people in Asia as nothing short of food of the gods. Soybeans are very high in protein, contain a heart-nourishing oil containing some omega-3 fatty acids, and contain isoflavones, phytochemicals with hormonelike effects that protect both men and women from certain forms of cancer. Difficult to digest in their dried form, the Asian culture discovered many ways to process soybeans in order to prepare them in ways that can be easily assimilated and enjoyed. Traditional forms of soy processing include miso, soy sauce, and tamari for seasoning and soy milk, tofu, and tempeh. Asian cuisine also enjoys the flavor and benefit of fresh soybeans in a dish called *edamame*, steamed fresh soybeans in their pods, tossed lightly with salt.

Fava Bean Stew with Summer Greens

With dark, leafy greens to ensure sufficient amounts of iron, calcium, folic acid, and fiber and the rich, creamy fava beans cooked with artichokes and a bit of olive oil, we'll finally achieve the complexion we all crave—smooth, line-free, moist, flawless. ▪ MAKES ABOUT 4 SERVINGS

1 pound fresh fava beans, in their pods

1 tablespoon extra-virgin olive oil

1 red onion, cut into thin half-moon slices

2 globe artichokes

Juice of 1 lemon

Grated zest of 1 lemon

Sea salt

Generous pinch dried basil

1 cup spring or filtered water

¼ cup mirin

1 small bunch dark leafy greens, rinsed, left whole

Shell the fava beans by trimming the tips, pressing open the seams of the pods, and gently pulling the beans out. Bring ½ inch of water to a boil over medium heat. Add the beans and boil until tender, about 10 minutes. Drain and set aside.

Place the olive oil in a deep skillet. Add the onion and place over medium heat. Sauté the onion until limp, about 5 minutes.

Trim the artichokes by removing the toughest outer leaves. Trim off the stems. With a small scissors, trim the top edges off each leaf. Finally, cut off the top half of the artichokes and discard. Trim away any dark leaves at the base. Carefully pull out the sharp inner leaves and the hairy choke in the center, taking care not to damage the heart of the artichoke. Split the artichokes, from top to bottom, into 4 equal wedges. Toss with lemon juice to prevent discoloration.

Add the lemon zest, a generous pinch of sea salt, basil, water, and mirin to the onion mixture. Stir well. Top with artichoke pieces, cover, and reduce heat to low. Simmer until tender, about 25 minutes. Stir in the fava beans, season to taste with salt, and simmer another 10 minutes.

Finely slice greens and stir into fava bean mixture. Cover, turn off heat, and allow to stand, covered, until greens just wilt, about 3 minutes. Stir gently to combine and serve immediately.

Veggie-Bean Ragout

Long-cooked beans and root vegetables give us deep-rooted strength and stamina. The beans provide us with a gentle protein that will keep us strong and nourished without overworking the liver and kidneys. And when the liver and kidneys are relaxed and happy, we have a line-free face; we don't look washed out and pallid. ▪ MAKES 4 TO 6 SERVINGS

1-inch piece kombu

1 sweet onion, halved lengthwise, each half cut into 4 wedges

2 cups 1-inch cubes winter squash

1 cup 1-inch pieces green cabbage

1 parsnip, cut into 1-inch irregular chunks

1 carrot, cut into 1-inch irregular chunks

1 cup cooked baby lima beans (see Note, below)

Grated zest of 1 lemon

¼ cup mirin

Soy sauce

Small handful fresh parsley, minced

Place the kombu on the bottom of a deep pot. Layer the vegetables in the pot in the order listed, ending with the beans on top. Add the lemon zest and mirin and enough spring or filtered water to just cover the bottom of the pot. Sprinkle lightly with soy sauce, cover, and bring to a boil over medium–low heat. Reduce heat to low and simmer until vegetables are just tender, but not mushy, about 35 minutes. Season to taste with soy sauce and cook, uncovered, until any remaining liquid has been absorbed into the dish. Gently stir in parsley and serve.

NOTE To cook baby lima beans, soak them for 2 hours in lightly salted water to prevent the skins from splitting. Drain the beans and cook in 3 cups fresh water with a 1-inch piece kombu until just tender, about 45 minutes. Drain away any remaining liquid.

Black Soybean Succotash

Succotash is a traditional bean dish, introduced to early settlers by Native Americans. Most likely, a local shell bean was used, but I'm using black soybeans as the base of the dish. Reputed to restore reproductive health, from the reduction of PMS symptoms to cooling off those annoying hot flashes that make menopause such a splendid experience, these lovely, sweet beans cool and relax the body. The sautéed vegetables give us vitality; the corn moisturizes the skin. We feel great and look even better. ■ MAKES 4 TO 5 SERVINGS

1 cup black soybeans, rinsed well, towel dried

1-inch piece kombu

3 cups spring or filtered water

2 tablespoons extra-virgin olive oil

1 yellow onion, diced

Soy sauce

1 teaspoon mirin

2 cups fresh or frozen corn kernels

1 cup plain soy milk

3 to 4 tablespoons fresh chives, finely minced

2 to 3 cherry tomatoes, thinly sliced, for garnish

Heat a dry skillet over medium heat and pan-toast the black soybeans. At first, they'll wrinkle and then they'll split open, revealing a white line through the bean. When about 80 percent of the beans are split and they are quite fragrant, transfer them to a pressure cooker. Work the kombu to the bottom of the pot, under the beans. Add the water and bring to a boil, uncovered, over medium heat. Allow to boil, uncovered, for 5 minutes. Seal the pressure cooker and bring to full pressure. Reduce heat to low and cook beans for 45 minutes. Remove from heat and allow pressure to reduce naturally.

Add the oil and onion to a deep skillet and place over medium heat. When the onion begins to sizzle sauté with a dash of soy sauce until limp, about 2 minutes. Stir in the mirin, corn, and soy milk, season lightly with soy sauce, reduce heat to low, and cook until slightly thickened, 5 to 7 minutes. Stir in the cooked black soybeans and simmer 1 to 2 minutes, just to develop the flavor. Remove from heat and stir in the chives. Serve garnished with the cherry tomato slices.

Mediterranean Bean Salad

There is nothing healthier than the Mediterranean approach to eating. Moderate, varied, and rich in taste and texture, these wholesome eating patterns have a lesson for all of us. With roots solidly in the use of vegetables, with meat and dairy as side dishes, if used at all, these traditions offer us a healthful and delicious style of eating that can last a lifetime. ■ MAKES 4 TO 5 SERVINGS

1-inch piece kombu

1 cup chickpeas, rinsed, brought to a boil, soaked 1 hour, drained

3 cups spring or filtered water

1 small head curly endive or bitter lettuce

2 to 3 tablespoons extra-virgin olive oil

1 clove garlic, thinly sliced

1 small red onion, cut into thin half-moons

Sea salt

Grated zest of 1 lemon

5 to 6 crimini mushrooms, brushed free of dirt, thinly sliced

1 carrot, cut into thin matchstick pieces

½ cup thin matchstick pieces daikon

2 teaspoons mirin

1 small cucumber, cut into thin half-moon slices

2 to 3 red radishes, thinly sliced

½ cup minced flat-leaf parsley

2 to 3 tablespoons balsamic vinegar

Juice of 1 lemon

Place the kombu on the bottom of a pressure cooker and top with the chickpeas. Add the water and bring to a boil, uncovered, over medium heat. Boil for 5 minutes. Seal lid and bring to full pressure. Reduce heat to low and cook for 45 minutes. Remove from heat and allow pressure to reduce naturally. Drain the beans and set aside.

Rinse and dry the endive very well. Slice finely and arrange on a platter. Chill thoroughly.

Add the oil and garlic to a skillet and place over medium heat. Cook the garlic until golden, strain from the oil, and discard. (This will give your dish the essence of garlic flavor without the strong energy associated with it.) Add the onion to skillet and sauté with a pinch of salt until limp, about 2 minutes. Stir in the lemon zest, mushrooms, and a pinch of salt and sauté until the mushrooms begin to release their juices into the pan. Stir in the carrot, daikon, and mirin. Season to taste with salt, reduce heat to low, and simmer, covered, until carrot is tender, about 7 minutes. Stir in cooked chickpeas and cook, uncovered, until any remaining liquid has been absorbed into the dish.

Remove from heat and mix in the cucumbers, radishes, parsley, vinegar, and lemon juice. Stir gently to combine. Spoon the chickpea mixture onto chilled endive and serve immediately.

Flageolets with Bitter Greens

Flageolets are small, pale-green to white beans, with a delicate flavor and gentle energy. Cooling and relaxing to the body, these mild-mannered beans can aid the body in releasing tension. Add to them the bitter greens, which can aid in relaxing the liver (so we're more patient and calm), and you have created a warm salad that leaves you looking refreshed and calm, always a good face to show the world. ■ MAKES 3 TO 4 SERVINGS

1-inch piece kombu

⅔ cup dried flageolets, rinsed well

3 cups spring or filtered water

2 to 3 tablespoons extra-virgin olive oil

1 small leek, split lengthwise, rinsed well, thinly sliced on the diagonal

Soy sauce

2 teaspoons mirin

1 red bell pepper, roasted over an open flame, peeled, seeded, thinly sliced
   (see Note, page 178)

1 medium head escarole, rinsed very well, coarsely shredded

Lemon wedges, for garnish

Place the kombu on the bottom of a heavy pot and top with the beans. Add the water and bring to a boil, uncovered, over medium heat. Reduce heat to low, cover, and cook the beans until tender, about 50 minutes. Drain away any remaining liquid and set aside.

Add the oil and leek to a deep skillet and place over medium heat. When the leek begins to sizzle, add a dash of soy sauce and the mirin. Sauté until the leek is limp, about 3 minutes. Stir in the bell pepper. Stir in the escarole, season lightly with soy sauce, and sauté until quite limp, about 5 minutes. Stir in the cooked beans to combine. Transfer to a serving platter and serve garnished with lemon wedges.

Tempeh-Stuffed Acorn Squash

Richly flavored stuffed squash is a great beauty food. Not just enjoyed during holiday seasons, this dish can make us look as sweet as sugarplums. Baking squash draws the sugars to the surface, making it sweetly satisfying. The sautéed filling has moisture-rich vegetables and protein-packed, fermented tempeh. Put it all together for a dish that relaxes the spleen, pancreas, and stomach, making us graceful under pressure with the strength of protein to make us walk tall.

■ MAKES 4 SERVINGS

2 medium acorn squash

1 tablespoon extra-virgin olive oil

½ sweet onion, diced

Soy sauce

1 small carrot, diced

1 to 2 stalks celery, diced

½ cup pine nuts, lightly pan-toasted

8 ounces tempeh, coarsely crumbled

¼ cup barley malt

¼ cup brown rice syrup

1 teaspoon light olive oil

Small handful fresh, minced parsley, for garnish

Preheat oven to 400F (205C). Line a baking sheet with sides with parchment paper.

Split the acorn squash in half lengthwise and remove seeds and stringy pulp. Turn, cut side down, and slice enough off the bottom of each half to create a flat edge. Place, cut side up, on the baking sheet, cover loosely with foil and bake for 15 minutes. Remove from oven, uncover, and set aside.

Place the extra-virgin olive oil and onion in a skillet over medium heat. When the onion begins to sizzle, add a dash of soy sauce and sauté until limp, 1 to 2 minutes. Add the carrot, celery, and a dash of soy sauce and sauté 2 minutes more. Stir in the pine nuts and tempeh, season lightly with soy sauce, reduce heat to low, and cook, stirring frequently, for 5 to 7 minutes. Remove from heat and stir well.

Spoon the tempeh filling generously into the bowl of each squash. Whisk together the barley malt, rice syrup and light olive oil. Spoon generously over filling and cut sides of squash. Cover loosely with foil and bake for 15 minutes. Remove cover and drizzle barley malt mixture over squash. Bake 20 to 25 minutes, or until the squash is quite tender and the filling is browned. Serve hot.

Fresh Soybean Salad

Lightly dressed in a spicy sesame dressing, this light vegetable and soy salad is a delicate side dish with a twist—sweet, tender cantaloupe. Strengthening, sweet root vegetables are the backdrops for the light energy of the fresh soybeans, creating a cooling, yet vitalizing dish, packed with nutrients and moisture for a flawless complexion. Try to find fresh organic soybeans whenever possible, as the nonorganic versions may be grown from genetically modified seeds. ■ MAKES 3 TO 4 SERVINGS

Sea salt

1 cup shelled fresh or frozen green soybeans

1 small parsnip, diced

1 small carrot, diced

1 cup diced daikon

SESAME DRESSING

1 tablespoon toasted sesame oil

1 to 2 fresh small red chile peppers, seeded, minced

Grated zest of 1 lemon

1 tablespoon brown rice syrup

2 teaspoons brown rice vinegar

1 tablespoon soy sauce

¼ cantaloupe, rind removed, seeded, diced

2 stalks celery, diced

Juice of 1 lemon

¼ cup black sesame seeds, pan-toasted, for garnish

Bring a pot of water to a boil. Add a pinch of salt and the soybeans. Boil the soybeans until just tender, about 5 minutes. Do not overcook. (They should be greener than before cooking.) Drain the soybeans and transfer to a bowl, saving the water. In the same water, cook the parsnip until just tender, about 4 minutes. Drain and add to soybeans. In the same water, cook the carrot until just tender, 3 to 4 minutes, drain, and add to the soybeans and parsnip. In the same water, cook the daikon 2 to 3 minutes, drain, and stir into soybeans.

Make the dressing: In a wok or deep skillet, heat the oil over medium heat. Add the chile and lemon zest and sauté for 1 minute. Add the rice syrup, rice vinegar, and soy sauce and stir well to combine.

Remove from heat and stir in the cooked vegetables and soybeans, along with the cantaloupe, celery, and lemon juice. Stir until ingredients are well coated. Serve warm, garnished with the black sesame seeds.

Tofu with Pureed Broccoli Sauce

Tofu is packed with protein and isoflavones, low in fat and calories, rich in calcium and vitamin D, cooling to the body, and able to release tension in the body. So why all the fuss? Simple. Tofu has a texture unfamiliar to the American palate, and while we may climb mountains, we're not all that adventurous with our food. I suggest, however, that you give it a go. All the magical properties attributed to tofu are true. ■ MAKES ABOUT 4 SERVINGS

3 tablespoons soy sauce

2 teaspoons mirin

Spring or filtered water

About 3 tablespoons light sesame oil

1 (about 1-pound) block extra-firm tofu, sliced into ½-inch-thick slabs

PUREED BROCCOLI SAUCE

2 to 3 tablespoons light sesame oil

5 to 6 slices fresh ginger

1 cup cooked white navy beans

3 to 4 broccoli stalks, broken into florets, stems peeled and sliced

Mirin

Sea salt

1 red bell pepper, roasted over an open flame, peeled, seeded, diced (see
  Note, page 178), for garnish

Mix the soy sauce and mirin in a shallow baking dish. Lay the tofu slices in marinade and add enough water to cover and allow to stand 5 to 7 minutes. Heat enough sesame oil to generously cover the bottom of a skillet over medium heat. Drain the marinade off the tofu. Pan-fry the tofu until golden, about 2 minutes on each side. Place fried tofu in a warm oven while making the sauce.

Make the sauce: Heat the oil and ginger in a small saucepan over medium to infuse the oil with ginger flavor, 2 to 3 minutes. Strain the ginger from oil and set aside to cool slightly. Stir in the cooked beans.

Steam the broccoli florets and stems just until bright green, about 4 minutes. Drain and transfer to a food processor. Add the beans, oil, mirin, and sea salt to taste. Puree until smooth.

To serve, lay tofu slices on a platter and spoon broccoli sauce over top. Garnish with the bell pepper. Serve warm.

Tofu Caponata

Caponata is a zesty Mediterranean relish that is traditionally served as a side dish. I'm turning it into a main course by adding tiny fried tofu cubes, which add protein while cooling and relaxing the body. Served on a bed of delicately bitter frisée (curly endive) to relax the liver, this caponata releases tension in the body, helps to eliminate furrows between the brows, and cool hot tempers.

■ MAKES 5 TO 6 SERVINGS

About 4 tablespoons extra-virgin olive oil

2 stalks celery, diced

Sea salt

1 to 2 zucchini, diced

1 to 2 yellow summer squash, diced

1 carrot, diced

1 red onion, diced

1 tablespoon brown rice syrup

2 teaspoons balsamic vinegar

½ cup minced, pitted, oil-cured black olives

½ cup pine nuts, lightly pan-toasted

2 to 3 tablespoons drained capers

Light olive oil, for frying

6 ounces extra-firm tofu, cut into ¼-inch cubes

Juice of 1 lemon

1 to 2 small bunches frisée, rinsed well, coarsely diced

Heat 1 tablespoon of the extra-virgin olive oil in a skillet over medium heat. Add the celery and a pinch of salt and sauté 1 to 2 minutes. With a slotted spoon, remove celery to a mixing bowl. Add another 1 tablespoon of the oil to the skillet. Add the zucchini and a pinch of salt and sauté 2 to 3 minutes. Remove to the mixing bowl with a slotted spoon. If needed, add a little more oil to the skillet, add the yellow squash and a pinch of salt, and sauté 2 to 3 minutes. Remove to a mixing bowl. Finally, heat a little more oil in the skillet. Add the carrot and a pinch of salt and sauté 3 to 4 minutes. Transfer to the mixing bowl. Gently mix to combine the vegetables.

Heat another 1 tablespoon oil in the skillet and add the onion and sauté until limp, about 3 minutes. Stir in the rice syrup and balsamic vinegar and cook, stirring, 2 to 3 minutes more. Stir cooked vegetables into the onion mixture. Turn off heat and stir in olives, pine nuts, and capers. Transfer to a mixing bowl and set aside.

Heat 2 inches of oil in a saucepan over medium heat. Add the tofu, a few cubes at a time, and fry until golden. Remove from oil and drain on paper. Stir the tofu into vegetable mixture. Add the lemon juice and stir to combine.

To serve, arrange the frisée on a serving platter and mound caponata on top. Serve at room temperature.

Maria's Tofu and Pasta Pie

Not so much a recipe for beauty as a recipe by a beautiful woman. Fitting for this book, I thought. My godmother (and aunt) is one of the most intelligent, independent, creative, compassionate, and generous women to walk this earth, and if that doesn't make you beautiful, I can't imagine what will. ■ MAKES 8 TO 10 SERVINGS

CRUST

2½ cups whole-wheat pastry flour

Generous pinch sea salt

½ cup light olive oil

About 2 tablespoons spring or filtered water

FILLING

2 tablespoons plus ¼ cup extra-virgin olive oil

1 medium yellow onion, diced

Sea salt

2 cups pasta, such as rotelle, fusilli, rotini, or penne

3 red bell peppers, roasted over an open flame, peeled, seeded, diced (see
  Note, page 178)

1 teaspoon dried basil

1 pound firm tofu

5 to 6 leaves of broccoli rabe or kale, lightly steamed, diced

8 ounces shredded nondairy soy mozzarella

1 cup strained, diced tomatoes

Preheat the oven to 400F (205C) and lightly oil a 9-inch springform cake pan.

Make the dough for the crust: Combine the flour and salt in a bowl. Cut in the oil until it is the texture of wet sand. Slowly add water until dough just gathers together. Knead a few times to pull dough into a ball. Cover with a damp towel and set aside.

Make the filling: Place the 2 tablespoons oil, onions, and a pinch of salt in a skillet over medium heat. When they begin to sizzle, sauté for 1 minute. Reduce heat to medium-low and cook, stirring frequently, until the onion begins to brown.

Bring a pot of water to a boil and cook the pasta, with no salt, until 80 percent done. Drain, but do not rinse, and set aside.

Stir the bell pepper into the onion, season lightly with salt and add the basil. Sauté 2 minutes more.

Crumble the tofu with the ¼ cup oil, diced broccoli rabe, and salt to taste. Set aside.

To assemble, divide the dough into 2 pieces, two-thirds for the bottom crust, one-third for the top crust. Roll out the bottom crust between 2 sheets of parchment into a round that will reach up the sides of the springform pan, with a bit of excess to hang over the sides. Fit the bottom crust in the pan, without stretching the dough.

Layer half of the soy cheese, sautéed onion and pepper, tofu mixture, and diced tomatoes with all the pasta. Then layer the remaining diced tomatoes, tofu, onion and pepper, and soy cheese. Roll out the top crust and fit over the filling. Pull the overhang of the bottom crust up over the top crust and crimp to seal. With a sharp knife, make a few slits in the top crust to allow steam to escape. Lightly brush the top crust with a little olive oil.

Bake for 55 to 60 minutes, or until the crust is golden and the filling is hot and bubbling. Remove from oven and allow to stand for 10 minutes before releasing the sides of the pan. Slice into wedges and serve hot.

Tofu and Wild-Mushroom Bread Pudding

Making our creamy sauce from tofu, we cool and relax the body, get great protein for strength and achieve the smooth, rich texture we crave. The shiitake mush-rooms remove tightness in the muscles, nourish the kidneys, and help us digest the richness of the dish. The result? We get the tastes we crave, so we're satisfied and won't "eat around" our desires. Plus, our bodies and faces are relaxed and line-free. ▪ MAKES 6 TO 8 SERVINGS

3 tablespoons extra-virgin olive oil

4 to 5 shallots, thinly sliced

Sea salt

8 to 10 dried shiitake mushrooms, soaked until soft, stems removed, thinly
sliced

6 ounces oyster mushrooms, thinly sliced

8 to 10 crimini mushrooms, thinly sliced

3 portobello mushrooms, thinly sliced

2 tablespoons minced fresh basil

2 tablespoons minced fresh parsley

1 teaspoon minced fresh thyme

1 (about 1-pound) block firm tofu

1 cup plain soy milk

1 teaspoon baking powder

6 cups 1-inch cubes whole-grain sourdough bread, crusts removed

½ cup whole-wheat bread crumbs

¼ cup nondairy soy parmesan cheese

Preheat oven to 350F (175C) and lightly oil a 9-inch-square glass baking dish.

Place the oil and shallots and a pinch of salt in a skillet, over medium heat. Sauté the shallots until limp, about 2 minutes. Stir in the shiitake mushrooms and sauté for 1 minute. Add remaining mushrooms, season lightly with salt, and sauté until they begin to release their juices into the pan. Stir in the basil, parsley, and thyme, stir well, and continue cooking, stirring frequently, until the mushrooms are tender and beginning to brown, about 10 minutes. Remove from heat and set aside.

Combine the tofu, soy milk, and baking powder in a food processor. Season lightly with salt and puree until smooth. Transfer to a mixing bowl and fold in the bread cubes. Stir in the mushroom mixture and spoon evenly into prepared dish. Mix the bread crumbs and soy cheese together and sprinkle over top of the bread pudding.

Bake 50 to 60 minutes, or until browned at the edges and set in the center. Remove from oven and allow to set for 15 minutes before serving.

Marinated Tofu Stir-fry

Simple, elegant, and lovely are words usually used to describe the classic looks we all desire. And to achieve that cool beauty we need to make appropriate food choices. With tofu and mushrooms to relieve tight muscles, a bit of oil for moist skin and hair, fiber-rich vegetables for easy digestion, and brown rice to balance the whole act, this dish does it all and leaves us looking elegant and lovely.

■ MAKES 4 TO 6 SERVINGS

> 1 (about 1-pound) block extra-firm tofu, cut into 1-inch cubes
>
> Spring or filtered water
>
> About 4 tablespoons soy sauce
>
> About 1 tablespoon fresh ginger juice (see Note, page 201)
>
> About 1 tablespoon mirin
>
> Yellow cornmeal
>
> 6 tablespoons light sesame oil
>
> 1 red onion, cut into thin half-moon slices
>
> 2 to 3 dried shiitake mushrooms, soaked until soft, stems removed, thinly sliced
>
> 1 carrot, cut into thin matchstick pieces
>
> 2 teaspoons mirin
>
> 2 cups cooked brown basmati rice
>
> 2 to 3 fresh scallions, thinly sliced on the diagonal
>
> Brown rice vinegar

Place the tofu in a shallow baking dish and add enough water to cover. Stir in the soy sauce until the color of an amber beer. Add the ginger juice and mirin to taste and marinate the tofu for 15 to 20 minutes. Drain the tofu.

Dredge the tofu in cornmeal. Heat about 5 tablespoons of the oil in a skillet and cook tofu, turning on all sides, until golden brown and crispy. Drain on paper towels and set aside.

Wipe out the skillet and heat the remaining 1 tablespoon oil over medium heat. Add the onion and a dash of soy sauce and sauté, until limp, about 2 minutes. Add the mushrooms and sauté for 2 minutes. Stir in the carrot and sauté for 1 minute. Add the mirin and stir well. Top the vegetables with the rice, season lightly with soy sauce, and add enough water to just cover the bottom of the skillet. Reduce heat to low and simmer for 5 to 7 minutes. Remove from heat, stir in the fried tofu, scallions, and a generous dash of rice vinegar. Serve hot.

Crispy Tempeh with Sweet Mustard Sauce

Serving richly flavored tempeh on a bed of lightly stir-fried veggies, rich in moisture, nourishes our parched skin and hair. Just think, no tight faces, dried-out wrinkling, or split ends. Just deep strength, a flawless complexion, and hair that's your crowning glory. ■ MAKES 4 TO 5 SERVINGS

Light sesame oil

8 ounces tempeh, cut into 1-inch triangles

2 teaspoons toasted sesame oil

1 small red onion, cut into thin half-moon slices

Sea salt

1 carrot, cut into thin matchstick pieces

1 to 2 stalks celery, thinly sliced on the diagonal

1 bunch watercress, rinsed well, coarsely diced

SWEET MUSTARD SAUCE

1 cup apple juice

2 tablespoons stone-ground mustard

1 tablespoon brown rice syrup

2 teaspoons soy sauce

1 teaspoon kuzu, dissolved in 2 tablespoons cold water

Heat enough light sesame oil to cover the bottom of a skillet over medium heat. Add the tempeh and pan-fry, turning to brown on both sides. Drain on paper towels.

Wipe out the skillet and heat the toasted sesame oil. Add the onion and a pinch of salt and sauté until limp, about 2 minutes. Stir in the carrot and celery, season lightly with salt, and sauté for 2 to 3 minutes. Finally, stir in the watercress, cover, and turn off heat. Allow watercress to steam for 2 minutes. Stir well and arrange the vegetables on a serving platter.

Make mustard sauce: Combine the juice, mustard, rice syrup, and soy sauce in a saucepan. Cook over low heat until warmed through. Stir in the dissolved kuzu and cook, stirring, until the mixture thickens and clears, about 3 minutes. Remove from heat and stir the tempeh into the sauce.

To serve, spoon the tempeh and sauce over top of the vegetables. Serve hot.

Asian Coleslaw with Fried Tempeh

When we lightly fry foods, we create a satisfying energy that helps us to eat less, so we don't get heavy and lethargic from overeating. Lightly cooked, mild vegetables, like cabbage, plus cucumbers, with a bit of spice from radish, balances our bodies' quest for moisture to nourish our skin and hair without overworking our kidneys, which creates a pale, washed-out look. ■ MAKES 4 TO 5 SERVINGS

5 to 6 tablespoons light sesame oil

8 ounces tempeh, cut into ½-inch cubes

2 cups spring or filtered water

1-inch piece kombu

1 teaspoon soy sauce

½ head green cabbage, finely shredded

1 carrot, cut into fine matchstick pieces

1 small cucumber, cut into thin half-moon slices

SESAME VINAIGRETTE

¼ cup light sesame oil

2 teaspoons soy sauce

2 teaspoons brown rice syrup

½ teaspoon crushed red pepper

2 tablespoons brown rice vinegar

1 cup minced fresh parsley

Heat the sesame oil in a skillet over medium heat. Add the tempeh and pan-fry, turning to brown on all sides. Combine the tempeh with water, kombu, and soy sauce in a saucepan over medium heat. Bring to a boil, uncovered. Reduce heat to low and simmer 5 to 7 minutes. Strain out the tempeh and discard broth. Set aside.

Bring a pot of water to a boil and blanch the cabbage for 1 minute. Drain and transfer to a mixing bowl. Blanch the carrot for 1 minute, drain, and mix in with cabbage. Mix in the cucumber. Gently mix in tempeh cubes.

Prepare the dressing: Warm the sesame oil, soy sauce, rice syrup, and red pepper over low heat for 3 to 4 minutes. Remove from heat and whisk in the rice vinegar.

To serve, gently mix the dressing and parsley into tempeh and vegetable mixture. Serve warm.

Perky Pickles and
Cute Condiments

There are two "food groups" in whole-foods cooking that are often neglected, considered by many to be "just another thing to do." They seem to encompass the smallest details. It is, however, in these details that we make our own personal balance within our diet. These two types of cooking are quite traditional, allowing us to make our own judgment calls within more broad-based cooking. Achieving everything from improving digestion to influencing the quality of our blood to helping us battle muscle tension and fatigue, pickles and condiments are invaluable to our health.

Pickles are not all that familiar to most Americans, except when served as garlic dill pickles on the side of a hot pastrami sandwich. But in fact, pickling was developed as a way to preserve food during the winter when vegetables would become scarce. Even meat and fish were pickled to prevent spoilage. And while Asian cuisine elevated pickling to something of an art form, every culture pickled, from sauerkraut to pickled green tomatoes, even pickled fruit.

What's this got to do with your looks? As you may recall, we discussed earlier how intestinal function has a direct influence over the condition of our hair; if it's too dry, so are the intestines; too oily and the intestines are congested with protein and fat buildup; graying hair indicates that the intestines are struggling to assimilate minerals. Pickled foods, particularly vegetables, introduce friendly bacteria into the intestines, promoting healthy flora so that digestion is regular and smooth, giving you the strong, lustrous, problem-free hair you crave.

Condiments, on the other hand, are something of a wonder in their power over our health. The use of condiments can balance you in so many ways. Simple to make, most condiments include some form of salt, which is the vehicle that draws the balance of the nutrients in the recipe deep into the body. This factor alone makes these seemingly little details quite powerful for us. Influencing the quality of our blood, improving kidney function, relaxing the liver, opening the spleen, or regulating blood sugars, condiments can improve the quality of our complexion, removing spots, dots, blotches, not to mention puffiness or dark circles under our eyes.

Condiments and pickles are powerful. With pickles, a mere tablespoon of pickled food each day will yield the results you seek and with condiments, you need just a touch here and there, sprinkled lightly on grain or vegetable dishes, to sense almost immediate changes in how you feel.

A tip before the recipes: Wash vegetables very well before pickling, as any dirt left on them may cause them to spoil during the pickling process. You'll end up with a jar filled with moldy, sour veggies.

While there are recipes here, and of course, making your own condiments and pickles ensures that the quality of them is superior, you can purchase most of them in natural foods stores when you just can't seem to get it together to prepare them. But make them for yourself sometime; it's amazing to see the power in the details of life.

Asian-Style Pickled Vegetables

Known in Asian cuisine as tsukemono, this simple pickling process can be used for any vegetable. This combination, daikon and cucumber, is one of my favorites. Cooling to the body, it can aid in relieving muscle tension, while the daikon also works on removing any congestion building up in the intestinal tract. The result is a relaxed body, with a head of shiny hair. ▪ MAKES 4 TO 6 SERVINGS

1 cup very thin daikon slices

½ cucumber, cut into very thin half-moon slices

½ teaspoon sea salt

Juice of 1 lemon

1 teaspoon umeboshi vinegar

Generous pinch shi-chi-mi or chile powder

Mix the daikon and cucumber together in a small bowl and add the salt. Rub the salt into the vegetables with your fingers and let stand for 5 minutes. Toss the vegetables with the remaining ingredients, mixing well. Cover loosely and set aside to pickle for 10 to 12 hours, stirring occasionally. These pickles will keep for about 3 days after pickling, stored in an airtight container in the refrigerator.

Red Radish Pickles

This quick and easy pickle is amazingly delicious. Lightly sweet and spicy, it aids the body in breaking down accumulated fat and protein buildup, making it as efficient as it is beautiful. ▪ MAKES 6 TO 8 SERVINGS

¼ cup brown rice vinegar

¼ cup umeboshi vinegar

1 tablespoon brown rice syrup

2 teaspoons finely minced fresh ginger

2 cups thinly sliced red radishes

Whisk the vinegars, rice syrup, and ginger together in a small bowl. Spoon over the radishes and mix well. Set aside, stirring occasionally, for about 2 hours before serving. These pickles are fragile and will only keep, refrigerated, for a couple of days.

Pressed Salad

Quite traditional in whole-foods cooking, this quick pickle is the best of both worlds: the freshness of a raw salad, but lightly pressed and pickled to ease digestion. The combination packs a moisture punch for our parched skin and hair.

■ MAKES 3 TO 4 SERVINGS

> 5 to 6 leaves Chinese cabbage, finely shredded
>
> ½ cucumber, unpeeled, very thinly sliced on the diagonal
>
> 3 to 4 red radishes, very thinly sliced
>
> 2 to 3 fresh scallions, very thinly sliced on the diagonal
>
> 1 orange, peeled, very thinly sliced
>
> 3 tablespoons umeboshi vinegar
>
> 2 tablespoons balsamic vinegar

Mix all the vegetables and orange in a bowl. Add the vinegars and rub the vegetables through your fingers as you mix to introduce the salt into the surface of the ingredients. As you mix, they will begin to wilt and release their fluid into the bowl. Place a plate on top of the salad and a light weight on top of the plate to press the salad. Press for 20 to 30 minutes. Remove the plate from the salad and lightly squeeze to press any remaining fluid from the vegetables. Arrange on a platter and serve at room temperature or lightly chilled. This pickle will only keep for one or two days, refrigerated, before it wilts too much to be appetizing.

Garlic Miso Pickles

It doesn't get easier than this pickle—but patience must be a virtue, because you'll have to wait 30 days to enjoy it. But when you do, these lightly spicy, quite salty pickles are great for improving our overall vitality and strength. And we always look our best when we can stand in our power.

1 pound barley miso

2 to 3 cloves garlic, peeled, halved

1 onion, cut into ¼-inch-thick half-moon slices

6 to 8 (⅛-inch-thick) diagonal carrot slices

Press the miso into a glass jar. Using a skewer or chopstick, push the garlic halves into the miso, distributing them throughout the jar. Carefully, push the onion and carrot completely into the miso, so they are covered, taking care that they don't touch, as that can make them spoil. Cover the jar with cheesecloth, securing it with a rubber band around the rim. Set aside in a cool place, but not the refrigerator, for 30 days before taking any pickles from the miso. You may leave the vegetables in the miso for as long as you like, but 30 days is the minimum.

When removing veggies from the miso, they will need to be rinsed and soaked in water for 30 minutes before consuming, as they will be quite salty. You'll need only a piece or two to achieve your goals with this powerful pickle.

You may continue to use this miso for years, replacing veggies in the miso as many times as you'd like. Just remember that if you are not actually pickling in the miso, keep it refrigerated until ready to pickle again.

Condiments

Sesame Salt (Gomashio)

Two simple ingredients come together to create a powerfully energizing condiment that can be used several times a week to battle fatigue or maintain vitality. Traditionally sprinkled on grain, this condiment balances the blood chemistry, making the blood more alkaline than acid, a much better environment for maintaining good health. And we look our best when we're feeling balanced.
■ MAKES ABOUT ½ CUP

1 teaspoon sea salt
6 tablespoons black or tan sesame seeds

Heat a dry stainless steel skillet over medium heat. Pan-toast the salt, stirring constantly, until its strong aroma dissipates and it turns a light gray color. Transfer the toasted salt to a suribachi (an Asian ceramic bowl, lined with ridges, for grinding) and grind with a wooden pestle until the salt becomes a fine powder.

In the same skillet, over medium-low heat, pan-toast the sesame seeds until fragrant and slightly puffed, about 5 minutes. Transfer to the suribachi, on top of the salt, and grind until the seeds are about half-broken. Cool completely before transferring to a dry glass jar. Sealed tightly, in the pantry, this condiment will keep for about a month.

For the best balance, use this condiment in ½-teaspoon quantities.

Pumpkin Seed–Shiso Powder

This hearty, delicately sour condiment is one of your liver's best pals. The mild character of the pumpkin seeds relaxes the middle organs—spleen, pancreas, and stomach—while the sour shiso powder opens and relaxes the liver. The result is a relaxed, stress-free face, with no little furrows between your lovely brows. It beats botox injections. ■ MAKES ABOUT ¾ CUP

1 cup pumpkin seeds (pepitas)

2 teaspoons shiso powder

Heat a dry skillet over medium heat. Add the pumpkin seeds and pan-toast until fragrant and slightly puffed and golden, 5 to 7 minutes. Transfer the seeds to a suribachi (an Asian ceramic bowl, lined with ridges, for grinding) and begin to grind until the seeds begin to break open. Add the shiso powder and continue to grind together until a coarse powder forms. Cool completely before transferring to a dry, glass jar. Sealed tightly, this condiment will keep for about a month.

This condiment is best served on grains or in vegetable dishes. For the best balance, use in ½-teaspoon quantities.

Miso-Scallion Relish

Richly flavored, sautéed in oil, and light in energy, this condiment is great for relaxing and lifting your spirits. A delicate condiment, it adds richness and moisture to our skin and hair, while preventing the lethargic energy that can make us look and feel washed out. ▪ MAKES ABOUT 6 SERVINGS

2 teaspoons light sesame oil

1 bunch fresh scallions, finely diced

1½ tablespoons barley miso, dissolved in a small amount of warm water

Heat the oil in a small skillet over medium heat. Add the scallions and sauté for about 1 minute. Stir in the dissolved miso and add enough water to cover the ingredients. Reduce heat to medium-low and cook, uncovered, until the mixture naturally thickens and the scallions begin to caramelize, about 20 minutes. Serve a dollop over grain.

This condiment will only keep about 2 days, refrigerated. Reheat before using.

Natto with Scallions and Mustard

Natto is a traditional Japanese condiment made from fermented soybeans. Completely unique in taste and texture, natto defies description, and for most Americans, is an acquired taste. Even though you may have to work a bit to be dazzled by this strongly flavored food, it's worth it. Its effect on the quality of our blood and resulting vitality is immeasurable. ■ MAKES ABOUT ½ CUP

> **4 ounces frozen natto, thawed (see Note below)**
> **3 to 4 fresh scallions, finely diced**
> **½ teaspoon soy sauce**
> **1 teaspoon stone-ground mustard**

Transfer the natto to a small mixing bowl. Mix in the remaining ingredients, and using wooden chopsticks, whisk briskly. The natto will take on a texture similar to mozzarella cheese, with stretchy "strings" developing.

The average serving size is 1 teaspoon. Serve with nori strips, over cooked brown rice, or as the filling in nori maki.

NOTE Natto is purchased in natural-food stores or Japanese markets and is sold frozen. Keep frozen until use, as natto will continue to ferment if left thawed for more than 24 hours. Unused portions of a container may be refrozen for later use, with no compromise to the integrity of the natto.

Delectable Desserts

Surprised to find a dessert chapter in a book about natural beauty? Good. Surprises are great for circulating blood to the face. Seriously, while we all love dessert, we have learned to fear this most delicious part of the meal. And with the large amounts of fat and simple sugars in modern desserts, we *should* be afraid, *very* afraid. But what if I told you that it didn't have to be that way—that you could have your cake and eat it, to coin a phrase?

When it comes to beauty, we look our best when we're relaxed, which is where dessert comes in. Dessert can serve us in our quest for health. In whole foods cuisine, all the foods we use have a purpose; nothing is arbitrary, from the most elaborate main course to the humble sprig of parsley being used for garnish.

The body responds most dramatically to sweet flavor. It satisfies, relaxes, centers; it makes us happy; it leaves us feeling sated and contented. Think about it: It's unlikely that you ever find yourself absolutely craving another heart of lettuce salad when you're stressed, upset, happy, or want to celebrate. We don't create birthday stews or wedding onion rings. We celebrate with sweet cakes.

So what's the deal with dessert? Is it good for us or bad? It can be either, depending on what's in it. Desserts made with white flour, sugar, heavy cream, milk, eggs, colorings, and artifical flavorings will, at the very least, make us fat and lethargic, with mood swings that can rival the highest roller coasters. In addition, they don't really satisfy our taste for sweet; we think they do, but the reality is that these kinds of foods only make us want more of them. Because they are made of simple sugar and white flour, these foods send your glycemic index into such a tailspin that the only way to stability is to load up on more sugar. The real answer is to break the pattern of sugar highs and lows. That's not always easy, but it's the only answer. The best news is that giving up simple sugar doesn't condemn you to a grim existence without sweet treats in your future. It's just a matter of switching around a few ingredients and making healthier choices. You will still create delicious, satisfying desserts, but you will create them with ingredients that leave you in charge of when you eat them, not the other way around.

But the news gets better. If the desserts you are choosing are of superior quality, made from fresh, whole ingredients—whole-grain flours and sweeteners, organic seasonal fruit, nuts and other healthy items—then dessert takes on a whole new face, so to speak. Not only does it satisfy your sweet desires, but there's no compromise to your health in the process. Is it a bit more work to eat healthier treats, since you'll need to make most of them? Yes, of course. Is your health worth the effort? It is, if you want to eat dessert and live to tell about it.

I've saved the best news for last. If you enjoy a small dessert frequently, several times a week, you will actually consume less food. As our bodies strive to relax, we eat more food, subconsciously deducing that being full will open our bodies and relax them. The reality is that more food, even good-quality food, makes the body work harder, leaving it tired. If, on the other hand, our diets contain regular portions of something sweet, we eat less food; we have fewer cravings; we stop binge eating. The body feels relaxed and satisfied with less, making it easier to achieve and maintain our ideal weight.

Healthy Sweets

When it comes to dessert creation, I am unwilling to compromise on health, quality of ingredients, taste, and appeal. So how do we create enjoyable, healthful desserts? How do we bake light, moist cakes and muffins; flaky pie crusts and pastries; rich, chewy cookies? How do we avoid creating those whole foods desserts that are healthy but have a bland taste and dry texture?

It is learning, through experimentation and practice, how the ingredients you are using will work together. Remember that the ingredients may change, but the techniques remain the same. For example, conventional cakes are light, moist, and springy to the touch due to the combination of eggs, white flour, milk, and sugar, as well as intense whipping during the mixing process (imparting air into the batter for that familiar light texture). Whole-grain–based cakes will never yield exactly that texture. However, you *can* create a light, moist cake that has full-bodied taste and texture.

The most important thing to remember is that desserts should always taste like an indulgence with a bit of oil for butteriness, nuts for rich taste, and sweetener for satisfaction. Attention to detail and superior quality ingredients will create the lush flavor in desserts that you are looking for and will enjoy for a lifetime.

INGREDIENTS AND TECHNIQUES
Flours

I use only whole-wheat pastry flour when baking cakes, cookies, pie crusts, pastries, muffins, tortes, cupcakes, or other baked treats. It is a finer grind of flour, ground from a softer strain of wheat, quite different from regular whole-wheat flour (which is great for breads, but not desserts), and creates a lighter end-product.

Fat Sources

To create moist textures in your pastries, you need a fat or fat substitute. Conventional baked goods rely on milk, cream, eggs, butter, margarine, or artificial fat additives. Since I choose not to cook with any of those foods, viable alternatives had to be discovered. My past experience has shown corn oil to be the clear winner, imparting a buttery flavor unsurpassed by other oils and creating a tender crumb and flavorful pastry. Canola oil was a distant second choice, because the cultivation of rapeseed (the source of canola oil) can be depleting to the soil and my environmentalist soul had a hard time sacrificing the planet for dessert. However, with the advent of corn oil from genetically modified corn, canola oil grew in its appeal, because there is canola oil pressed from nongenetically modified seeds, and the resulting desserts were very nice. The moral dilemma had reached epic proportions for me. The answer came when I was looking through some old family recipes and found a pound cake that was made with light olive oil instead of butter. I had a culinary epiphany and began to scour old Italian cookbooks and found that light olive oil is used with great frequency in desserts. I worked through all the basics—pie crusts, cookies, pastry, cakes, even pancakes—and the results are so dreamy that I can't wait for you to give these recipes a try. The flavor is rich and buttery, with delectable moisture and an exquisite golden color. Substitute olive oil in any recipe where you are using corn or canola oil for spectacular results.

For those of you who wish to eliminate fat altogether in your baking, I have found that applesauce or pureed poached pears work nicely to create a moist cake. Other liquids in the recipe will need to be adjusted to accommodate the liquid in the fruit.

Flavorings

Depth of flavor is where dessert really soars. Conventional desserts have the benefit of lots of fat, dairy products, and artificial ingredients to impart rich taste. Healthful desserts must be more creative to deliver satisfaction.

Always purchase pure vanilla, almond, and other extracts, not artificially flavored ones, for all your desserts. Don't ignore the sweet and hot spices. Adding a hot spice such as hot chile pepper or black pepper may be just the right touch in a chocolate cookie or cake. A little vinegar or lemon juice can bring a recipe to life and bring out its sweetness.

Adding citrus zest to a recipe is a sensational way to add depth of flavor to desserts. The zest is the colored part of the outer skin of lemons, oranges, and other citrus fruits and adds a tangy zip to fruit compotes, sauces, cakes, pastries, and puddings. Because zest only has a mild sweet zing to it, you can use it as you desire.

Egg Substitutes

Eggs are used in desserts for two reasons, to leaven and to bind. There are a couple of alternatives to eggs in dessert making. For leavening, you may add 1 teaspoon of nonaluminum baking powder for every egg in the recipe.

In recipes where eggs act as binders, I have substituted 1 teaspoon kuzu or arrowroot dissolved in a little water for each egg and have been quite successful. For custards or flans, a combination of agar flakes and kuzu have proved most satisfying in providing a firm, creamy pudding. Usually 1 tablespoon each of kuzu and agar is enough to yield the firmest, creamiest custards.

Dairy Substitutes

With the popularity of soy milk soaring, it should be no surprise to discover that it is a great milk substitute. Another option for milk, especially for custards and cream fillings, is amasake, a sweet, fermented rice milk. You can also try my favorite product from Eden Foods, Eden Rice and Soy Blend, which combines soy milk with fermented rice milk (amasake).

Nuts

Nuts are a wonderful addition to healthful desserts for many reasons. The fat content in nuts gives desserts a rich, distinctive flavor and their texture adds an interestingly appealing crunch. To get the best flavor from nuts, lightly roast them before use: the lower the oven temperature, the more flavorful the nuts. For instance, I roast pecans at 275F (135C) for about 20 minutes to bring forth their delicate flavor. A high roasting temperature will result in a bitter flavor. Pan roasting nuts on the stovetop yields a more delicate flavor and is the method I prefer, except with pecans and hazelnuts, which do better in the oven.

Sweeteners

I've saved the best for last. Sugar will kill us, literally, so what's the alternative? The best-quality sweeteners I have found are grain-based. Barley malt and brown rice syrup are the sweeteners I choose. These are mostly complex carbohydrates, not simple sugars, so they are released into the blood slowly, providing fuel for the body instead of creating the ups and downs we experience when we eat simple sugars. They are simply whole grains, inoculated with a fermenting agent and then cooked until they reduce to a syrup.

Rice syrup yields a delicate sweetness that is very satisfying, with no aftertaste. It is the perfect sweetener for most cakes, pastries, cookies, and puddings. Barley malt has a stronger flavor, much like molasses, so I reserve it for desserts that complement that kind of taste, like spice cakes, carrot cakes, pumpkin pie, and caramel sauces.

I rarely use honey, maple syrup, or fruit sweeteners, again, because they are simple sugars, and also because they have such a strong sweet taste, which can overpower the other dessert flavors.

Techniques

Now I know that most pastry chefs will tell you that you must always sift flour before mixing with other ingredients to create air in the batter, not once or twice, but three times. When I worked as a pastry chef, I was tutored by an incredibly talented chef, who broke all the rules. He never sifted; he never mixed wet and dry ingredients separately. And he made the most wonderful temptations, but that was his way. Over the years I have made my own discoveries, as you will, but here is what I know from my own experiences: Sifting is not a necessary step. Instead, I mix the dry ingredients and whisk them briskly. With the wet ingredients, I mix the oil and sweetener into the dry ingredients and then slowly stir in the remaining wet ingredients, until I achieve the texture I desire, taking care to avoid overmixing, which will remove air from the batter, leaving you with a heavy, tough dough. Also, remember that whole grain loves moisture, so overmixing will cause the flour to saturate itself, making it impossible to rise and remain tender.

Assemble all the ingredients before you begin to bake. Preheat the oven and prepare the baking pans before you begin. This will allow you to work quickly. You want to mix the batter and bake it. You don't want it sitting for several minutes while you prepare the pans and heat the oven. Letting the batter sit for several minutes will result in a heavy end-product.

When mixing ingredients, use pastry knives, forks, spoons, anything but your hands. The oil from your skin will coat the flour and can create a tough, spongy dough. Handle the dough only when necessary, as the recipe requires. Don't knead dough unless the recipe requires it; and when it does, don't over-knead, or under-knead. Inexperienced bakers would do well to follow recipes to the letter until certain techniques are mastered and you develop a "feel" for the doughs and batters. With practice, you will develop an intuition for baking.

Grilled Pears with Minted Glaze

Desserts like this one, with sticky, seemingly rich glazes will satisfy our desire for sweet indulgences without any compromise to our digestion and without landing heavily on our hips. ▪ MAKES 4 SERVINGS

> 2 large, firm-ripe pears
> 2 teaspoons light olive oil
> Sea salt
> ¼ cup brown rice syrup
> 1 teaspoon finely minced fresh mint leaves
> 2 teaspoons grated lemon zest
> Fresh berries, for garnish

Preheat a grill pan to medium-high. Peel and halve the pears. With a melon baller or a small spoon, carefully remove the cores. Leaving the stem end intact, slice each pear half into ⅛-inch-thick slices almost to the stem end. Lightly brush the pear with oil, taking care to cover the cut edges. Sprinkle a pinch of salt over each half.

Gently press the pear halves onto the hot pan, fanning the slices. Cook until tender and deeply marked, about 3 minutes. Turn the halves by sliding a spatula under the pear, from the stem side. Cook until marked, again, about 3 minutes. Transfer pear halves to individual serving plates.

To prepare a glaze, combine the rice syrup, mint leaves, and lemon zest in a saucepan. Cook over medium heat just until the mixture foams. Spoon the glaze over each pear half and garnish with a few fresh berries.

Gingered Carrot Cake

Carrot cake is a traditional favorite, moist, sweet, hearty, and smothered with a creamy frosting. Veggie-based desserts can be good for you. Made from whole-grain flour and sweeteners with organic carrots, light oil, and nuts, this dessert satisfies without compromise. And with the rich caramel glaze, you'll never miss the cream cheese, and neither will your thighs. ▪ MAKES 8 TO 10 SERVINGS

GINGERED CARROT CAKE

1 cup pecan pieces

3 cups whole-wheat pastry flour

1 tablespoon baking powder

¼ teaspoon sea salt

1 teaspoon powdered ginger

1 teaspoon ground cinnamon

2½ cups grated carrots

½ cup unsweetened applesauce

½ cup light olive oil

½ cup brown rice syrup

1 teaspoon pure vanilla extract

½ to ⅔ cup Eden Rice & Soy Blend or vanilla soy milk

ORANGE CARAMEL GLAZE

¼ cup Eden Rice & Soy Blend or vanilla soy milk

⅔ cup brown rice syrup

2 tablespoons barley malt

Grated zest of 1 orange

Orange slices, for garnish

To make the cake: Preheat oven to 275F (135C) and spread the pecans on a baking sheet. Bake about 15 minutes, or until fragrant. Cool slightly and coarsely dice. Set aside.

Lightly oil and flour a 10-inch bundt pan. Increase the oven temperature to 325F (165C).

Combine the flour, baking powder, salt, and spices in a mixing bowl. Whisk briskly. Stir in the carrots, applesauce, oil, syrup, and vanilla. Slowly add enough Rice & Soy Blend to make a thick, spoonable batter. Spoon evenly into the prepared pan.

Bake 45 to 50 minutes, or until the center of the cake springs back to the touch or an inserted toothpick comes out clean. Allow the cake to cool in the pan for about 10 minutes before inverting onto a serving platter. Cool completely before glazing.

To make the glaze: Combine all ingredients in a saucepan and cook over medium heat until the mixture foams. Reduce heat to low and cook until the mixture reduces and thickens, 5 to 7 minutes. Immediately spoon over cake, repeating the glaze for several coats until the glaze is used up. Garnish with orange slices and serve.

Ruby Fruit Salad

Richly colored red fruits are simply lovely, and you'll look lovely after eating them. It's their potassium, succulent moisture, and low sugar content that make us shine. These jewels in the crown of the fruit kingdom nourish our skin by cleansing the kidneys with their astringent quality. ■ MAKES 4 TO 5 SERVINGS

¼ cup brown rice syrup

Grated zest of 1 orange

Juice of 1 orange

Juice of 1 lime

¼ cup mirin

¼ cup spring or filtered water

12 to 15 cherries, pitted, left whole

2 to 3 small red plums, halved, pitted, thinly sliced

½ pint strawberries, rinsed, halved

½ pint raspberries, rinsed

2 nectarines, halved, pitted, thinly sliced

Sea salt

Combine the rice syrup, orange zest and juice, lime juice, mirin, and water in a saucepan. Cook over medium heat until the mixture foams. Cool to warm, whisking to keep it loose.

Combine the fruit in a bowl. Sprinkle with 2 pinches of sea salt and gently mix in. Pour the syrup over the fruit mixture and gently fold in to coat the fruit. Cover and chill completely before serving.

Lemon Custard Cups

This dessert satisfies our craving for creamy puddings, our love affair with pastry, and our enchantment with desserts as beautiful as they are delicious. The rich flavor and light energy of this treat will leave you looking as delicious as you are, knowing that you're supporting your liver function as you nourish your sweet tooth. A relaxed liver means a line-free face and even-toned complexion.

■ MAKES 8 SERVINGS

LEMON CUSTARD

2 cups plain amasake or vanilla soy milk

2 tablespoons brown rice syrup

1 teaspoon pure vanilla extract

Grated zest of 1 lemon

Pinch sea salt

2 tablespoons kuzu, dissolved in 6 tablespoons cold water

Juice of 1 lemon

PASTRY CUPS

4 sheets fresh or frozen phyllo, thawed if frozen

Light olive oil

¼ to ½ cup plain bread crumbs

About ½ cup fresh seasonal berries, for garnish

To prepare the custard: Combine the amasake, rice syrup, vanilla, lemon zest, and salt in a saucepan. Warm through over low heat. Stir in the dissolved kuzu and cook, stirring, until the mixture thickens, about 3 minutes. Remove from heat and whisk in the lemon juice. Transfer custard to a heat-resistant bowl and cover with plastic wrap to prevent a "skin" from forming.

Preheat the oven to 375F (190C) and lightly oil 8 cups of a standard muffin pan.

Stack the phyllo sheets on a dry work surface. Slice phyllo into 6 (4-inch) squares. Press 1 phyllo square into each oiled cup. (Cover the remaining phyllo squares with a damp towel.) With a pastry brush, lightly oil each phyllo square and sprinkle with bread crumbs. Repeat with a second phyllo square in each cup, turning it at a different angle, oil, and sprinkle with bread crumbs. Repeat with a third square in each cup, turning, lightly oiling, but do not sprinkle with bread crumbs, making a total of 8 cups.

Bake about 6 minutes, or until golden and crispy. Transfer pan to a wire rack and cool cups completely in pan before gently lifting them out.

Just before serving, loosen custard with a whisk and generously fill each pastry cup. Garnish with fresh berries.

Coconut Macaroons

There's nothing quite like the paradox of macaroons, rich and decadent, with a decidedly light feel to them. And therein lies the art of this special treat. Each moist gem is unique, like a snowflake, light on the tongue but so sensual. The very thought of them makes you more beautiful, as you get that dreamy look in your eye, imagining the luxury of coconut and chocolate.

■ MAKES ABOUT 24 COOKIES

COCONUT MACAROONS

2½ cups unsweetened, shredded coconut

⅓ cup whole-wheat pastry flour

½ teaspoon baking powder

Pinch sea salt

⅓ cup brown rice syrup

½ teaspoon pure almond extract

⅔ cup almond milk

CHOCOLATE GLAZE

½ cup grain-sweetened, nondairy chocolate chips

2 to 3 tablespoons almond milk

2 teaspoons brown rice syrup

To make the macaroons: Preheat oven to 400F (205C). Line 2 baking sheets with parchment paper.

Combine all the ingredients for the cookies, mixing well. Set aside so the coconut can absorb the liquid, about 5 minutes. You should have a thick batter, but it will not be very cohesive. Drop the batter by teaspoonfuls onto baking sheets, and form into peaked cookies with your fingers. Bake about 20 minutes, or until the coconut begins to brown. Transfer to a wire rack to cool.

To make the glaze: Place the chocolate chips in a heat-resistant bowl. Combine the almond milk and rice syrup in a small saucepan and bring to a full boil. Pour over the chocolate and whisk until smooth and satinlike. Transfer to a plastic squeeze bottle.

Slip a piece of parchment paper under the wire rack. Moving in a zigzag direction, drizzle the cookies with the glaze. Allow to stand for a few minutes to set the glaze.

Gingerbread Cookies

There's something about gingerbread cookies; they're homey and cozy and oh so delicious. Here's another plus: the deep heat from the ginger and sparkling energy of the spices not only enliven the flavor of the cookie but vitalize us so we look great, line-free and fresh. ▪ MAKES 2 TO 3 DOZEN COOKIES

2 cups whole-wheat pastry flour

1 tablespoon unsweetened cocoa powder

2½ teaspoons powdered ginger

1 teaspoon ground cinnamon

¼ teaspoon ground cloves

1 teaspoon baking powder

Generous pinch sea salt

¼ cup light olive oil

⅔ cup brown rice syrup

1 teaspoon pure vanilla extract

¼ to ½ cup Eden Rice & Soy Blend or vanilla soy milk

Nuts and raisins, for decoration (optional)

Combine the dry ingredients in a bowl and whisk briskly to combine. Stir in the oil, rice syrup, and vanilla. Slowly add enough Rice & Soy Blend to create a smooth, stiff dough. The dough should come together, but not be too sticky or too crumbly. Turn out onto a lightly floured surface and knead a few times. Divide dough into 4 pieces. Wrap 3 pieces in plastic wrap.

Preheat oven to 350F (175C). Line 2 baking sheets with parchment paper. Lightly re-flour your work surface and rolling pin. Roll out 1 piece of dough to ⅛-inch thickness. Cut into desired shapes with cookie cutters or a round glass. Decorate if desired with nuts and raisins. Transfer to baking sheets, using a spatula. Repeat with remaining dough pieces, re-rolling the scraps.

Bake 10 to 12 minutes, or until the edges begin to brown. Let the cookies cool on the pans until firm; transfer to wire racks to cool completely.

VARIATION Brush with warmed brown rice syrup for a glaze.

Lemon Thumbprints

Small, chewy cookies are a great dessert choice when you are concerned about your appearance. Here's why: Soft flour products are easier to digest, so the body is less stressed, and when the body is relaxed, we look younger. Soft cookies have a delicacy that satisfies easily, so we tend not to overindulge.

■ MAKES ABOUT 3 DOZEN

    2½ cups whole-wheat pastry flour

    1½ teaspoons baking powder

    Generous pinch sea salt

    Grated zest of 1 lemon

    ½ cup light olive oil

    ½ cup brown rice syrup

    1 teaspoon pure vanilla extract

    Juice of ½ lemon

    ¼ to ½ cup Eden Rice & Soy Blend or vanilla soy milk

    About ½ cup unsweetened raspberry, strawberry, or apricot preserves

Preheat oven to 325F (165C). Line 2 baking sheets with parchment paper.

Combine the flour, baking powder, salt, and lemon zest in a mixing bowl. Whisk briskly to combine. Stir in the oil, rice syrup, vanilla, and lemon juice. Slowly mix in enough Rice & Soy Blend to form a soft, pliable dough.

Form dough into 1-inch balls and place on baking sheets about 1 inch apart. Using a damp finger, make a deep well in the center of each cookie. Spoon preserves into each well, filling generously.

Bake on the center rack 20 to 22 minutes, or until the cookies are just firm and lightly golden on the bottom,. Do not overbake or the cookies will get quite hard as they cool. Remove cookies from the oven and transfer immediately to wire racks to cool.

Amazing Sticky Buns

Nothing makes us feel more content in the morning than sticky buns. Gooey, rich, delicious, and oh, so relaxing. But can they be good for us? With whole-grain flour and sweeteners, we can have our sticky buns and not compromise our health. The pastry chef at the Essene Natural Market and Cafe in Philadelphia passed this wonderful recipe to me. ■ MAKES 12 STICKY BUNS

4 cups whole-wheat pastry flour

1 cup spring or filtered water

2 tablespoons active dry yeast

½ teaspoon sea salt

½ to 1 cup natural apple juice

⅓ cup brown rice syrup

⅛ cup light olive oil

2 sticks (1 cup) nondairy soy margarine, chilled

2¼ cups brown rice syrup

About 1 teaspoon ground cinnamon

⅔ to 1 cup pecan pieces, coarsely chopped

Place the flour in a mixing bowl. Warm the water through over low heat until lukewarm. Mix in the yeast and set aside for 15 minutes.

Mix the salt, ½ cup apple juice, rice syrup, and oil, along with the yeast mixture into the flour. Stir until the dough comes together, adding additional apple juice if needed, and the dough is no longer sticky. (You may need to sprinkle a bit of flour into the mixture to bring the dough to this state.) Cover dough with a dry towel and set aside in a warm place to rise until doubled in size, about 1 hour.

Punch down the dough to remove air. Turn the dough out onto a lightly floured surface. Roll out to flatten slightly. Slice 1 margarine stick into thin pieces and arrange on half the dough. Fold dough in half and roll out again. Slice remaining margarine into pieces and arrange on half the dough. Fold in half and roll out to flatten slightly. Repeat the folding and rolling process two more times.

Roll out dough to form a large rectangle that is about ⅛-inch thick. Drizzle dough with ¾ to 1 cup of the rice syrup and spread over dough. Sprinkle lightly with cinnamon. Roll, jelly-roll style, into a long cylinder.

Generously oil a muffin pan. Spoon the remaining rice syrup evenly into the muffin cups and top with the pecan pieces. Slice the dough roll into 12 equal pieces and place in muffin cups. Cover with a towel and place in a warm area to rise until doubled in size, about 45 minutes.

Meanwhile, preheat oven to 350F (175C). Bake 25 to 30 minutes, or until the buns are a rich golden brown. Remove buns from muffin pans while still warm.

Apple Pudding with Lemon Glaze

Steamed puddings satisfy many needs. Moist and succulent, they make us feel relaxed. Richly flavored, we're happy with a smaller serving, so our hips will thank us. They're steamed, not baked, so we can have the flour we desire but digest it more easily, not exhausting our digestive tract, which means we never look our age. ■ MAKES 8 TO 10 SERVINGS

APPLE PUDDING

2 cups whole-wheat pastry flour

2 teaspoons baking powder

½ teaspoon ground cinnamon

¼ teaspoon grated nutmeg

½ teaspoon powdered ginger

Generous pinch sea salt

¼ cup light olive oil

½ cup brown rice syrup

1 teaspoon pure vanilla extract

¾ to 1 cup Eden Rice & Soy Blend

1 Granny Smith apple, peeled, cored, diced

Grated zest of 1 lemon

½ cup unsweetened, shredded coconut

½ cup minced, lightly toasted pecans (see page 281)

LEMON GLAZE

Grated zest of 1 lemon

¼ cup brown rice syrup

Lemon slices, for garnish

To make the pudding: Lightly oil a 1-quart pudding basin and its lid.

Combine the flour, baking powder, spices, and salt in a mixing bowl. Mix in the oil, rice syrup, and vanilla. Slowly mix in the Rice & Soy Blend to create a smooth, spoonable cake batter. Fold in the apple, lemon zest, coconut, and pecans. Spoon into prepared pudding basin. Seal the lid and place in a pot large enough to hold the basin with a generous amount of space around it. Add water to the pot to half cover the pudding basin. Cover the pot and bring to a boil over medium heat. Reduce heat to low and simmer for 2 hours, adding more water to the pot after 1 hour, if necessary. The water level needs to be maintained to ensure the moistness of the pudding.

Carefully remove the pudding basin from the larger pot and set aside to cool for 10 minutes. Remove the basin lid and loosen the pudding from the sides, by gently running a knife around the rim. Place a plate over the pudding and invert the basin onto the plate. Remove the basin and set the pudding aside to cool completely.

To make the glaze: Heat the lemon zest and rice syrup over medium heat until it foams. Spoon the glaze over pudding, allowing it to run down the sides. Garnish with fresh lemon slices.

Chocolate Passion Drops

This recipe is an example of layering flavors in a recipe. The chile powder and black pepper accentuate the sweetness of the chocolate and give it a gentle punch. We never look better than when in the throes of chocolate passion.

■ MAKES 2 DOZEN

1⅓ cups whole-wheat pastry flour

¾ cup unsweetened cocoa powder

1 teaspoon baking powder

⅛ teaspoon sea salt

⅛ teaspoon freshly ground black pepper

⅛ teaspoon chile powder

¾ teaspoon ground cinnamon

¾ cup light olive oil

½ cup brown rice syrup

1 teaspoon pure vanilla extract

About 2 tablespoons Eden Rice & Soy Blend or vanilla soy milk

½ cup grain-sweetened, nondairy chocolate chips

CHOCOLATE-COCONUT TOPPING

3 tablespoons Eden Rice & Soy Blend or vanilla soy milk

1½ tablespoons brown rice syrup

½ cup grain-sweetened, nondairy chocolate chips

About ¼ cup unsweetened shredded coconut

Preheat oven to 350F (175C). Line 2 baking sheets with parchment paper. Combine the dry ingredients in a mixing bowl. Whisk to blend. Stir in the oil, rice syrup, and vanilla. Slowly add enough Rice & Soy Blend to make a soft, moldable dough.

Roll the dough into 1-inch balls. Place on prepared baking sheets. Bake 12 to 14 minutes; cookies should be set but still soft. Transfer cookies to a wire rack to cool.

To make the topping: Combine the Rice & Soy Blend and rice syrup in a small saucepan and bring to a boil over medium heat. Turn off heat and stir in the chocolate chips, stirring until smooth and satinlike. Dip the tops of the cookies in the chocolate mixture, then into the coconut.

Fruity Lattice Cobbler

People say that drinking red wine makes the French ageless. Well, it's true. It's not the alcohol; it's the rich, red color, the tannin. Any foods that are brightly colored, particularly red, will have the same effect on us as red wine, contributing to the ageless beauty of our skin. Puts a whole new spin on cherries, doesn't it?

■ MAKES 8 TO 10 SERVINGS

FILLING

4 cups fresh cherries, pitted

2 cups fresh raspberries

1 cup blueberries

2 tablespoons arrowroot

1 tablespoon light olive oil

½ cup FruitSource (granulated brown rice syrup and fruit)

Grated zest of 1 lemon

1 teaspoon pure vanilla extract

BISCUIT CRUST

2 cups whole-wheat pastry flour

1 teaspoon baking powder

Pinch sea salt

¼ cup light olive oil, plus oil for brushing

¼ cup brown rice syrup

½ to ⅔ cup Eden Rice & Soy Blend or vanilla soy milk

Preheat oven to 350F (175C). Lightly oil a 10-inch deep-dish pie plate.

To make the filling: Combine the fruit in a mixing bowl. Stir in the arrowroot, oil, FruitSource, lemon zest, and vanilla to coat the fruit. Spoon evenly into pie plate and set aside.

To make the crust: Combine the flour, baking powder, and salt in a food processor. Add the oil and rice syrup and pulse until they are incorporated into the flour mixture, about 45 times. Slowly add Rice & Soy Blend down the feed tube, pulsing, until the dough just gathers into a ball. Do not make the dough too sticky. Transfer dough to a lightly floured work surface and roll out to a ⅛-inch-thick round that is about an inch bigger than the pie plate. Cut the round into 1-inch-wide strips.

To weave a lattice top, lay half the dough strips, evenly spaced, over the top of the fruit. Do not stretch the dough. Fold back every other strip to its midway point. Beginning at the fold, lay a strip at a 90-degree angle over the other strips. Unfold the strips, crossing the new one. Fold back the strips, alternate to the first ones, to the strip that is across. Lay another strip, evenly spaced, parallel to the cross strip. Continue in this pattern until you reach the edge of the pie plate. You will have latticed half the cobbler top. Repeat with balance of dough strips on the other half of the cobbler. Let any excess dough hang over the edge of the pie plate. After the top is complete, cut the overhanging dough away, with a sharp knife, flush with the edge of the pie plate.

Brush the lattice top lightly with olive oil, cover loosely with foil, and bake, on a baking pan (to catch any juices that may cook over) for 25 minutes. Remove foil tent and bake another 25 to 30 minutes, or until the biscuit top is lightly browned and the fruit is bubbling.

Pecan Fruit Crisp

Fruit crisps are simple to make, casual to serve, versatile, and oh, so satisfying. Baking the fruit gentles the effect of sugar on the blood, the topping satisfies our desire for flour, and the pecans add richness, without being heavy in the belly or on the hips. ■ MAKES 8 TO 10 SERVINGS

PECAN TOPPING

1 cup pecans

3 tablespoons whole-wheat pastry flour

½ teaspoon baking powder

¾ cup FruitSource (granulated brown rice syrup and fruit)

½ cup rolled oats

¼ cup light olive oil

FILLING

4 to 5 apples, Red or Golden Delicious or McIntosh

½ cup unsweetened dried cherries, soaked for 15 minutes

Generous pinch sea salt

2 tablespoons arrowroot

1 tablespoon light olive oil

3 tablespoons brown rice syrup

To make the topping: Preheat oven to 300F (150C). Spread the pecans on a baking sheet and bake about 15 minutes, or until fragrant. Cool slightly and coarsely mince. Set aside. Increase oven temperature to 350F (175C).

Combine the flour, baking powder, FruitSource, and oats in a food processor and pulse until a fine flour forms. Transfer to a mixing bowl and cut in oil until the mixture is the texture of wet sand. Stir in the pecans and set aside.

To make the filling: Peel, halve, and core the apples. Slice thinly. Drain the cherries, discarding the soaking water. Combine the apples, cherries, salt, arrowroot, oil, and rice syrup in a bowl and mix well to coat the fruit. Spoon fruit into a 10-inch deep-dish pie plate.

Cover fruit with the topping. Cover loosely with foil and bake 25 minutes. Remove foil and bake another 30 minutes, or until the topping is lightly browned and the fruit is soft.

Cherry-Pear Turnovers

Turnovers are a special dessert. Sparkling fruit filling is shrouded in a soft pastry dough, creating a richly flavored treat. The good news for our looks is that turnovers are small, so we can enjoy one without a lot of guilt. A small indulgence will prevent those digestively exhausting binges that leave us looking washed out and feeling lethargic. ■ MAKES 10 TURNOVERS

PASTRY

2 cups whole-wheat pastry flour

Generous pinch sea salt

1 teaspoon baking powder

1 to 2 tablespoons light olive oil

½ cup unsweetened applesauce

1 tablespoon brown rice syrup

1 teaspoon pure vanilla extract

Spring or filtered water

PEAR FILLING

2 cups diced peeled pears (3 to 4 pears)

½ cup unsweetened dried cherries, soaked for 15 minutes, drained, minced

1 vanilla bean, split lengthwise, pulp scraped

Grated zest of 1 lemon

¼ cup brown rice syrup

Spring or filtered water

TOPPING

Light olive oil, for brushing

½ cup sliced almonds

Preheat oven to 350F (175C). Line a baking sheet with parchment paper.

To make the pastry: Combine the flour, salt, and baking powder in a mixing bowl. Mix in the oil, applesauce, rice syrup, and vanilla. Dough will gather, but be dry. Slowly add water, by the tablespoonful, to create a soft dough, but not too much or the dough will be sticky. Wrap the dough in plastic wrap and set aside.

To make the filling: Combine the pears, cherries, vanilla bean pulp, zest, rice syrup, and water in a saucepan. Cook over medium–high heat, stirring constantly, until the water is absorbed, 7 to 10 minutes. Remove from heat and mash with a fork to create a chunky puree. Set aside to cool completely.

To assemble the turnovers: Divide the dough into 10 equal pieces. On a lightly floured surface, roll one piece into a 4-inch round. Re-wrap the remaining dough to keep it moist. Place a heaping spoonful of filling on the round. Moisten the edge of the round and fold the dough over filling, creating a semicircle. Seal by pressing a fork gently around the edge. Place the turnover on baking sheet. Repeat with remaining dough and filling. Brush each turnover lightly with oil and sprinkle with sliced almonds.

Bake 25 to 30 minutes, or until turnovers are golden brown.

Blueberry Upside-Down Cake

Brightly colored fruits and vegetables are great brain food; the richer the colors, the more mineral-rich the food. So dark greens, carrots, squash, red onions, melons, strawberries, raspberries, blackberries, and precious blueberries all aid in creating clear, focused thinking. Sweetly delicious, this cake is light, rich, and lights up our power to think, and we look great when we're smart. ■ MAKES ABOUT 4 SERVINGS

   4 tablespoons light olive oil

   ⅓ cup plus 3 tablespoons brown rice syrup

   1½ cups fresh blueberries, sorted, rinsed, drained

   Sea salt

   1 cup whole-wheat pastry flour

   1 teaspoon baking powder

   ¼ cup Eden Rice & Soy Blend or vanilla soy milk

Preheat oven to 350F (175C). Lightly oil a 1-quart (about 5½-inch) soufflé dish. Warm 1 tablespoon of the oil with 2 tablespoons rice syrup over low heat in a small saucepan until syrup thins, about 2 minutes. Spoon rice syrup mixture evenly over bottom of soufflé dish and sprinkle blueberries into the syrup. Sprinkle with a pinch of sea salt to sweeten the fruit. Set aside.

Combine the flour, baking powder, and a generous pinch of salt. Whisk briskly. Cut in the remaining oil and rice syrup. Slowly mix in Rice & Soy Blend to create a smooth, spoonable batter. Spoon batter evenly over berries, taking care not to disturb them.

Bake 40 to 45 minutes, or until the center of the cake springs back to the touch or a toothpick inserted in the center comes out clean. Immediately run a knife around the rim of the dish to loosen and invert the cake onto a platter. Spoon any topping that remains in the dish onto the cake. Serve warm.

Lemon–Poppy Seed Pound Cake

Nothing says "light" like lemon and nothing says "rich" like pound cake. But how do we create the satisfying, buttery texture of a pound cake without all the butterfat, which leaves us heavy, with oily skin and hair? Light olive oil, baby. Ever check out Italian women's skin? It's flawless, supple, line-free at most any age.

■ MAKES 8 TO 10 SERVINGS

LEMON–POPPY SEED POUND CAKE

2½ cups whole-wheat pastry flour

1 tablespoon baking powder

¼ teaspoon sea salt

Grated zest of 2 lemons

2 tablespoons poppy seeds

½ cup light olive oil

½ cup brown rice syrup

1 teaspoon pure vanilla extract

Juice of 2 lemons

½ to 1 cup Eden Rice & Soy Blend or vanilla soy milk

LEMON GLAZE

½ cup brown rice syrup

Grated zest of 1 lemon

To make the cake: Preheat oven to 325F (165C). Lightly oil and flour a 9 × 5-inch loaf pan.

Combine the flour, baking powder, salt, zest, and poppy seeds. Whisk briskly. Mix in the oil, rice syrup, vanilla, and lemon juice. Slowly add enough Rice & Soy Blend to create a smooth, spoonable batter. Spoon into prepared loaf pan.

Bake 35 to 40 minutes, or until the center of the loaf springs back to the touch or an inserted toothpick comes out clean. Remove from oven and allow to cool in the pan for 10 minutes. Run a sharp knife around the rim of the pan to loosen the cake and invert loaf onto a wire rack to cool completely.

To make the glaze: Heat the rice syrup and zest in a small saucepan over medium heat until it foams. Immediately spoon the glaze over the cake.

Chocolate Ginger Cake

Chocolate as a beauty food? Think about it. It's rich, smooth, and as satisfying as a food can get. However, chocolate as most of us know it is also full of sugar, additives, and saturated fats, so not so great. How can we enjoy this "food of the gods" and not pay the price? Choose a good quality, unsweetened, organic (when possible) chocolate and make the recipes you enjoy with the finest ingredients you can find. The richness of chocolate is incredibly satisfying to women, much more than to men. Why? Magnesium. When our magnesium levels are on an even keel, we may love chocolate, but just a taste will satisfy our desire.

■ MAKES 8 TO 10 SERVINGS

CHOCOLATE-GINGER CAKE

½ cup unsweetened cocoa powder, plus extra for dusting

2½ cups whole-wheat pastry flour

¼ teaspoon sea salt

1 tablespoon baking powder

½ cup unsweetened, shredded coconut

1 tablespoon powdered ginger

1 teaspoon ground cinnamon

½ cup light olive oil

⅔ cup brown rice syrup

1 teaspoon brown rice vinegar

1 teaspoon pure vanilla extract

1 to 1½ cups Eden Rice & Soy Blend or vanilla soy milk

CHOCOLATE GLAZE

¼ cup Eden Rice & Soy Blend or vanilla soy milk

3 tablespoons brown rice syrup

1 cup grain-sweetened, nondairy chocolate chips

To make the cake: Preheat oven to 350F (175C). Lightly oil a 10-inch bundt pan. Instead of flour, dust the pan with cocoa powder, so that the cake doesn't have white deposits on it.

Combine the cocoa powder, flour, salt, baking powder, coconut, and spices. Whisk briskly. Mix in the oil, rice syrup, vinegar, and vanilla. Slowly add enough Rice & Soy Blend to create a smooth, spoonable batter. Spoon evenly into the prepared pan.

Bake 35 to 40 minutes, or until the top of the cake springs back to the touch or an inserted toothpick comes out clean. Remove the cake from the oven and allow to stand for 10 minutes before inverting onto a platter. Allow to cool completely.

To make the glaze: Combine the Rice & Soy Blend and rice syrup in a saucepan and bring to a boil over medium heat. Turn off heat and stir in chocolate chips, stirring until smooth and satinlike. Immediately spoon a thin glaze over cake, allowing it to run down the sides. Allow to set 1 to 2 minutes and repeat with another layer of glaze, continuing until the cake is glazed as you like.

Vanilla Shortcake with Summer Fruit

This dessert has all the decadence with none of the guilt, made from whole natural ingredients, no sugar, no dairy fats—nothing but rich flavor, satisfyingly sweet and deliciously light. If our sweets are light and healthy but richly flavored, we're satisfied. When we're satisfied, we're not binging. And when we're not binging, we look and feel beautiful. ■ MAKES 8 TO 10 SERVINGS

VANILLA SHORTCAKE

2 cups whole-wheat pastry flour

2 teaspoons baking powder

Generous pinch sea salt

¼ cup light olive oil

¼ cup brown rice syrup

1 teaspoon pure vanilla extract

⅔ to 1 cup Eden Rice & Soy Blend or vanilla rice or soy milk

½ teaspoon umeboshi vinegar

FRUIT TOPPING

1 to 2 cups red grapes

1 cup raspberries

2 to 3 peaches, halved, pitted, thinly sliced

2 to 3 red plums, halved, pitted, thinly sliced

Grated zest of 1 lemon

Juice of 1 orange

Generous pinch sea salt

⅓ cup brown rice syrup

VANILLA CUSTARD

1 cup plain amasake

½ cup Eden Rice & Soy Blend or vanilla soy milk

1 vanilla bean, split lengthwise, pulp scraped, or 1 teaspoon pure vanilla extract

1 tablespoon kuzu, dissolved in 3 tablespoons cold water

To make the cake: Preheat oven to 375F (190C). Line a baking sheet with parchment.

Combine the flour, baking powder, and salt in a mixing bowl. Whisk briskly. Mix in the oil, rice syrup, and vanilla. Mix the ⅔ cup Rice & Soy Blend with vinegar (to simulate buttermilk) and stir into flour mixture. The dough should gather and be soft, but not sticky. Add additional Rice & Soy Blend if needed. Turn dough out onto a lightly floured surface and knead 6 times to gather the dough. Transfer to the baking sheet and form into an 8-inch round.

Bake 20 to 25 minutes, or until the top is lightly browned and a toothpick inserted comes out clean. Transfer cake to wire rack to cool.

To make the topping: Combine all the ingredients in a mixing bowl and stir to combine. Set aside to marinate for at least 30 minutes.

To make the custard: Combine the amasake, Rice & Soy Blend, and vanilla-bean pulp in a saucepan and warm through over low heat. Stir in dissolved kuzu and cook, stirring, until the mixture thickens, 3 to 4 minutes. Set aside to cool and thicken completely.

To serve, place the cake on a serving platter. Spoon fruit over top, mounding generously. Whisk custard to loosen and spoon over fruit. Another way to serve is to slice the cake into wedges, place a wedge on each individual dessert plate, and mound with fruit and a generous dollop of vanilla custard.

Spicy Pear Tarte Tatin

Upside-down cakes are so cozy and casual; their rustic look makes everyone relax and enjoy themselves. The spices and citrus zest nicely balance the sweet pears, gentling the sugars, so we can digest the pears as easily as the moist cake that cushions them. And when our tummy's in order, we look line-free and rested.
■ MAKES 6 TO 8 SERVINGS

FILLING

5 to 6 ripe, but firm pears, halved, cored, thinly sliced

Juice of 1 lemon

Pinch sea salt

¼ cup light olive oil

⅔ cup brown rice syrup

Pinch ground cinnamon

Generous pinch powdered ginger

Grated zest of 1 lemon

3 tablespoons raisins

CAKE

2 cups whole-wheat pastry flour

2 teaspoons baking powder

Generous pinch sea salt

¼ cup light olive oil

¼ cup brown rice syrup

½ to ⅔ cup Eden Rice & Soy Blend or vanilla soy milk

To make the filling: Toss the pears in the lemon juice and salt and allow to stand for 5 minutes. In a deep 10-inch, cast-iron skillet, combine the oil, rice syrup, spices, and lemon zest. Cook over medium-low heat until syrup thins, about 2 minutes. Drain pear slices and arrange in the skillet. Top the pears with the raisins and cook over low heat until dark and caramelized, about 15 minutes. Arrange in a decorative pattern on the skillet surface. Remove from heat.

Preheat oven to 325F (165C). To make the cake: Combine the flour, baking powder, and salt in a mixing bowl. Whisk briskly. Stir in the oil and rice syrup. Slowly mix in enough Rice & Soy Blend to create a smooth batter. Spoon the batter carefully over arranged pears to evenly cover.

Bake 35 to 40 minutes, or until the center of the cake springs back to the touch or an inserted toothpick comes out clean. Immediately run a sharp knife around the rim of the skillet to loosen the cake and invert it onto a platter. Carefully remove any fruit that is left in the skillet and replace it on the surface of the cake.

Remedies to Glow By

To maintain our health and a youthful, glowing appearance, as well as increase our odds for a long and vital life, nothing, nothing replaces our daily food choices in importance. Eating food appropriate for a human being, along with exercise and a positive attitude are our best bets for feeling and looking our best. Now and then, however, we need a helping hand, for an acute symptom, to get moving, to kick-start our healing process, or to feel more energized. For those moments, I present a few natural remedies—some brews and potions, if you will, to help to set your feet on the path to your glow. I don't recommend that you rely too heavily on these simple recipes—like using them in place of a healthy eating plan—but they just might be the ticket to get you going.

Both internal and external, these simple, natural remedies can help to relieve symptoms and alter problems—for the short haul—while your diet and lifestyle adjustments work on your long-term, natural radiance.

Carrot-Daikon Drink

This spicy, pungent tea is designed to help dissolve hardened fat deposits that have accumulated around various organs, making for sluggish function and lethargy—and as such, is a great kick-start for weight loss. Working deep in the body to restore balance, this drink works to dissolve the fat, while adding minerals to create strong blood quality. As hardened fat begins to break apart, the weight loss process can begin. For the best results, take this tea every other day for two weeks, then stop for two weeks, repeating again, if needed. If you have begun losing weight during the first round of this drink, wait longer than two weeks before repeating again for another two weeks. Let nature, and life changes, do their job. ■ MAKES 1 SERVING

¼ cup finely grated carrot

¼ cup finely grated daikon

1 cup spring or filtered water

Splash soy sauce

⅓ sheet toasted sushi nori, shredded

⅓ umeboshi plum

Combine the grated vegetables with water in a saucepan and bring to a gentle boil, uncovered, over medium heat. Reduce heat to low and simmer 3 to 4 minutes. Add the soy sauce and simmer 2 to 3 minutes more. Stir in the nori and umeboshi plum and simmer 1 minute more. Drink the tea and eat the vegetables, while the tea is quite hot.

NOTE For a stronger tea, eliminate the nori and umeboshi plum, using only the carrot and daikon. It is more potent this way, so you cannot use this tea for as long a period of time. It'll make you feel tired, so be careful.

Adzuki Bean Tea

Puffy, swollen bags under the eyes indicate that the kidneys are becoming swollen and weak, unable to do their job, overcome by too much liquid, simple sugars, even fruit juices. These little jewellike beans, low in fat and high in potassium, are prized in Asian healing for their ability to restore the mineral balance in the blood and kidneys to efficient function. For best results, take this tea two to three times a week for about a month. You'll feel stronger, more vital, and your eyes will look fresh and rested each morning. ■ MAKES 1 SERVING

¼ cup adzuki beans, rinsed well

½-inch piece kombu

1 cup spring or filtered water

Place the beans, kombu, and water in a saucepan. Bring to a boil, uncovered, over medium heat. Reduce heat to low and simmer for about 30 minutes. Strain out beans and drink tea while hot.

NOTE You may continue cooking the beans in soups or stews.

Shiitake Tea

Dark circles under the eyes seem to be the plague of humanity. This is a sign that your kidneys need a boost. Dark circles mean that they are becoming constricted and dry (you probably have lower back pain, too), the result of too little liquid, too much salt, too much stress, and too much strenuous activity. When the kidneys are in this state, we don't even sleep well. This simple tea is designed to regulate kidney moisture, softening them so they can do their job efficiently. For the best results, drink this two to three times a week for about a month. Your body will feel stronger, yet relaxed, and you will rest better. And your dark circles will become just a dim memory. ■ MAKES 1 SERVING

1 dried shiitake mushroom

1 cup spring or filtered water

Splash soy sauce

Soak the shiitake mushroom in water until tender, about 20 minutes. Finely mince and place, with the soaking water, in a saucepan. Bring to boil, uncovered. Reduce heat to low and simmer for 10 to 15 minutes.

Add the soy sauce and simmer 2 to 3 minutes more. Drink the liquid and eat mushroom while hot.

NOTE This tea can also be quite effective in relaxing overall tension or tightness in various muscles of the body, particularly in the shoulders and legs.

Kombu Tea

Kombu has so many benefits in the body, it's hard to count them all. Good for fortifying blood quality, dissolving hardened animal fats, and restoring nervous system function, this simple tea has amazing restorative powers. Rich in keratin, this tea aids in the production of strong, lustrous hair. Kombu contains a substance called monosodium glutamic acid that aids in the breakdown of fat, internally, and as we know it, cellulite. It takes time, but it can work. For the best results, take this tea two to three times a week for about three weeks and then, once a week, for another month. After that, just a cup from time to time is enough. ■ MAKES 2 SERVINGS*

4-inch piece kombu
4 cups spring or filtered water

Place the kombu and water in a saucepan. Bring to a boil, covered. Reduce heat to low and simmer until the liquid reduces by half, 10 to 15 minutes. Remove kombu. Drink one cup while hot. You may reheat any remaining tea for another serving.

Daikon Tea

A mild diuretic you can make yourself, with none of the negative side effects associated with those powerful drugs. It's great for premenstrual fluid retention, swollen ankles and fingers, even puffy eyes. For fluid retention, take this tea once a day for three days, take five days off, then repeat if needed. Repeat for no more than three cycles. ■ MAKES 1 SERVING*

½ cup grated daikon

1 cup spring or filtered water

Splash soy sauce

Squeeze the daikon to extract the juice. Combine the juice with the water in a saucepan. Bring to a gentle boil over medium heat. Reduce heat to low, add the soy sauce, and simmer for 1 minute. Drink while hot.

Ume-Sho-Kuzu

This tea has a strengthening effect on our digestion. When digestion is efficient, we stand straight, have confidence, eat less and feel satisfied longer, suffer no lined, dry, chapped lips, and have a flatter tummy.

While you can take this tea any time that your tummy is a bit upset, its strength lies in the long-term change it makes in the environment of your intestines, improving digestion over time. For best results, take this tea three times a week for a month. After that, you can take this tea now and then for fortitude, or if you get an upset stomach. ▪ MAKES 1 SERVING

⅓ umeboshi plum, finely minced

1 cup spring or filtered water

Pinch sea salt

1 teaspoon kuzu, dissolved in 2 teaspoons cold water

Combine all the ingredients in a small saucepan. Cook, stirring constantly, over low heat until the mixture thickens and clears, about 3 minutes. Drink while hot.

Sweet Barley-Malt Kuzu

To rid our faces of those annoying little frown lines, we need to relax our liver and this simple, sweet-and-sour tea is just the ticket. The rising sweetness of the barley malt with the sour taste of lemon juice combine with alkalizing kuzu to refresh and open a tight, tired liver. ▪ MAKES 1 SERVING

1 cup spring or filtered water

1 teaspoon kuzu

1 tablespoon barley malt

2 teaspoons fresh lemon juice

Combine all ingredients in a saucepan, stirring to dissolve the kuzu. Cook over low heat, stirring constantly until the tea thickens and clears, about 3 minutes. Drink while hot.

NOTE Do not overcook or the lemon juice will turn bitter.

Our Outer Glow

The Body Scrub

The most amazing remedy in the world, and you don't have to cook a thing. This remedy activates circulation, promoting clear, soft skin, by helping the skin eliminate toxins from the body. If you take nothing else from this book—if you don't ever cook a vegetable—scrub your body. It will change your life, and you'll really glow.

Quarter fold a cotton washcloth (or use a cloth spa glove purchased from a pharmacy). Using hot water, wet the cloth and begin to scrub your body (without soap), rubbing gently with just the weight of your hand, until your skin turns pink all over. Start with your hands, rubbing palm and back, between your fingers, and work your way up your arms toward your chest. Next, rub your chest and back, but for women, avoid the breasts and for men and women, the genitals, but scrub your groin area. Work your way down your belly, scrub your buttocks, and then work your way down your legs, front and back, to your feet, scrubbing the tops of your feet, between your toes, and even the soles of your feet.

At first, you'll notice that your skin turns a mottled pink. As the body breaks down accumulated, hardened fats, your skin will turn a uniform, rosy pink in minutes.

One month of faithful scrubbing and you'll notice a new softness to your skin, and you'll be addicted. In about two months, you'll find that you no longer need moisturizer, that you don't have flaky shins or crusty heels. For the best results, scrub every day.

Ginger Compress

This relaxing compress aids the body in dissolving hardened fats, revives stagnant energy, and stimulates blood circulation, warming and energizing the body. Most commonly used on the lower back to relax and strengthen the kidneys, this simple remedy is incredibly vitalizing. Great for relieving water retention, tired eyes, swollen fingers, and stiff, aching muscles. Doing this helps you to look rested and refreshed to face the day.

1 gallon water

4- to 5-inch piece ginger

Bring the water to a boil. While the water is heating, grate ginger to create a tennis ball–sized mound. Reduce heat to low to stop the boiling. Place the ginger in a piece of cheesecloth or thin cotton. Wrap the ginger and tie in a knot. Squeeze the ginger sack into the hot water and place the sack in the water. Simmer for about 5 minutes; do not boil.

Lay a thin towel over the part of the body you are treating, for example, the lower back for treating the kidneys. Dip another towel in the hot water, wring out tightly, and lay over thin towel. Cover with yet another dry towel to keep in the heat. Change the ginger towel when it no longer feels hot. Repeat compress until skin turns bright pink.

You may do a ginger compress two to three times a week, as desired. You may use the ginger water two to three times, as long as you are careful not to boil it as you reheat it.

Since this compress is stimulating to the circulation, it is not generally recommended for use on people with serious conditions like cancer.

Salt and Malt Scrub

I love to do this scrub every spring. It's great for freshening the skin after a winter spent indoors. Lightly exfoliating, without being abrasive to the skin, the warm, wet salt removes dreary winter skin and the barley malt seals in moisture for supple, soft, ready-for-spring skin. Once a year is enough for this luxurious scrub, particularly if you're doing The Body Scrub (page 313) regularly.

2 pounds (at least) refined sea salt

2 pounds barley malt or honey

Take a hot shower and rinse the body very well. While still wet, rub generous handfuls of salt gently over your skin. Don't apply a lot of pressure, as you can damage the skin, just a gentle rub. Rinse well with warm water and again, while wet, rub a thin layer of barley malt over your skin. Rinse well, pat your newly moisturized skin dry, go out, and enjoy the warm spring air.

Kombu Bath

If you think kombu is effective in teas and in cooking, try this bath. Kombu has the ability to break down fat in foods—and us. This soothing bath results in smooth, soft skin and aids the body in breaking down our ever-present cellulite. While not a magical instant cure, over time you will see a difference in the texture of orange-peel skin.

3 (6-inch) pieces kombu

1 generous handful sea salt

Add the kombu and salt to the bathtub. Run a hot bath, as hot as is comfortable. Simply soak in the tub for 10 to 15 minutes. You may rub the kombu over your skin for smoothing if desired. Rinse well and pat your skin dry. For best results, try this bath once a week. You may reuse the kombu three times.

Facial Scrub

Gentle facial scrubs, without harsh chemicals, are quite nice. They feel great and they gently exfoliate the tender facial skin, without abrading the surface, causing more of the very damage you are trying to heal. This one is simple to make and doesn't leave your face tight and dry. Good for all skin types, this once-a-week scrub is heavenly.

2 tablespoons oat bran

2 tablespoons warm rice milk (not soy)

Mix the ingredients together to form a paste. Wet your face with warm water. Spread gently over the face, to the jaw line, avoiding the tender skin under your eyes. Massage cleanser gently into your skin, using circular motions, 2 to 3 minutes. Rinse with slightly warm water, at least 20 times to remove the scrub, and finish with a few cold rinses. Pat your face dry and apply your daily moisturizer.

Facial Dabs

These simple home brews are a great way to freshen your skin when it feels dull and dry, or a bit oily and shiny, or if you're going through a series of breakouts. Just dab these potions on your skin for a fresh face to carry through the day.

Oily Skin

Brew a strong cup of kukicha or black tea. Cool thoroughly. Using a fresh cotton ball, dab over the face (or just the oily areas). The drying, cooling nature of tea will help to balance your skin on the surface, while you work on the internal balance that will make this dab not necessary.

Dry Skin

Warm 1 cup whole milk (one of the few uses for dairy milk that I suggest). Using a fresh cotton ball, dab the warm milk over your skin, rinse a few times with warm water, and apply moisturizer. The fatty nature of the milk will help to make your skin feel soft, while you concentrate on diet and lifestyle changes that make it naturally soft and lush.

There's nothing like a cup of hot milk in your bath, during those dry winter months, to keep your skin soft and supple.

Blemishes

Calendula is an herb that is revered for its anti-inflammatory and healing properties. Chamomile is an herb known to relax our systems and balance upsets. Together, these two herbs can relieve the inflammation that is causing the breakouts, while balancing the skin, at least until you do it with your diet.

1 tablespoon dried calendula

1 tablespoon dried chamomile

1 cup boiled water

Add the herbs to the water and steep until cooled to room temperature. Do not cool in the refrigerator, as it will weaken the brew. Using a fresh cotton ball, dab this gentle herbal potion on the blemishes. Don't rinse. This brew will keep, refrigerated, for 5 days. You may use it chilled or at room temperature.

Scalp Massage

For dry hair only, this scalp massage can help to restore your mane to its former luster. Scalp massage can help to stimulate circulation to the scalp, opening the clogged follicles that contribute to dry hair. Rosemary is an herb with oils that warm and activate circulation and its aromatic nature causes its energy to rise in the body, stimulating the scalp.

Buy some rosemary oil from a natural-food store or herbal shop. Dab some on each fingertip and work your fingers through your hair to your scalp. Firmly massage the scalp, in circular motions, covering the entire head, working from the nape of the neck to the top, down the sides. Rub with only your fingertips, not your nails, as they can break the scalp or cause irritation.

For a treatment for the entire hair shaft, work rosemary oil from root to tip after your scalp massage. Wrap your head in plastic; the heat from your body will warm the oil and intensify the treatment. Wash and moisturize your hair as usual.

For the best result, massage your scalp before every shampoo and use the intense whole head treatment once a week until your diet and lifestyle changes reveal your naturally shining locks.

Sea Plant Soak

A great anti-bloating soak, use it during those times just before your menstruation when you might retain a bit of fluid. A normal state, as your hormones are shifting and adjusting to your cycle, this bloating is nonetheless uncomfortable. Sea plants are prized in many cultures for their balancing and detoxifying effects in the body, as well as their ability to break down accumulated fat in various organ systems. This mild bath can help to normalize the balance of fluids in the body. This is also a nice bath for when you simply want to detox a bit and freshen your skin.

1 cup loosely packed arame

Grated zest of 1 lemon

6 to 8 cups water

Combine all the ingredients in a large pot and bring to a boil, uncovered. Reduce heat to low and simmer until the liquid is quite dark, about 15 minutes. Strain out the sea plant and lemon zest, reserving the liquid.

Run a hot bath, as hot as is comfortable. Add the reserved arame water and soak for 10 to 15 minutes. Rinse your skin well with warm water and pat your skin dry.

This bath, since it draws, is not recommended for use during menstruation, as it can cause a heavy flow.

Tired Eyes Relief

Here's some relief for those moments when you look as tired as you feel, when your eyes are feeling itchy and irritated from too many hours on the computer or you wake up looking less than refreshed and feel just plain tired. Chamomile, known for its ability to relax and balance, is just perfect for infusing a bit of energy into red, tired eyes.

1 tablespoon dried chamomile

1 cup boiling water

Place the chamomile in a glass bowl and add the boiling water. Allow to steep at room temperature, about 20 minutes. Strain out chamomile and discard. Soak two fresh cotton balls and place over closed eyes. Relax with eye packs in place for 10 minutes. The scent and nature of the herb will do the trick to refresh your tired eyes.

For morning puffiness, try these same eye packs, but chill the brewed chamomile overnight. Soak fresh cotton balls in the cold brew and apply to your puffy eyes. Leave on for 10 minutes and voila!

Bibliography

These are the texts that have become invaluable to me, both in my daily life and work, and in the writing of this book. My deepest gratitude to the authors.

Benn Hurley, Judith. *Savoring the Day*. New York: William Morrow, 1997.

Kushi, Aveline and Wendy Esko. *Diet for Natural Beauty*. New York: Japan Publications, Inc., 1991.

Kushi, Michio. *How to See Your Health: The Book of Oriental Diagnosis*. New York: Japan Publications, Inc., 1980.

———. *Your Face Never Lies*. Garden City, NJ: Avery, 1983.

Lu, Henry C. *Chinese Natural Cures*. New York: Black Dog & Leventhal, Inc., 1994.

Ohsawa, Georges. *You Are All Sanpaku*. New York: Citadel, 1965.

———. *Zen Macrobiotics*. Los Angeles: Ohsawa Foundation, Inc., 1965.

Veith, Ilza. *The Yellow Emperor's Classic of Internal Medicine*. Berkeley, CA: University of California Press, 1949.

Weil, Andrew. *Eating Well for Optimum Health*. New York: Knopf, 2000.

Metric Conversion Charts

COMPARISON TO METRIC MEASURE

When You Know	Symbol	Multiply By	To Find	Symbol
teaspoons	tsp.	5.0	milliliters	ml
tablespoons	tbsp.	15.0	milliliters	ml
fluid ounces	fl. oz	30.0	milliliters	ml
cups	c	0.24	liters	l
pints	pt	0.47	liters	l
quarts	qt.	0.95	liters	l
ounces	oz.	28.0	grams	g
pounds	lb.	0.45	kilograms	kg
Fahrenheit	F	5/9 (after subtracting 32)	Celsius	C

LIQUID MEASURE TO MILLIMETERS

¼	teaspoon	=	1.25	milliliters
½	teaspoon	=	2.5	milliliters
¾	teaspoon	=	3.75	milliliters
1	teaspoon	=	5.0	milliliters
1-¼	teaspoons	=	6.25	milliliters
1-½	teaspoons	=	7.5	milliliters
1-¾	teaspoons	=	8.75	milliliters
2	teaspoons	=	10.0	milliliters
1	tablespoon	=	15.0	milliliters
2	tablespoons	=	30.0	milliliters

FAHRENHEIT TO CELCIUS

F	C
200-205	95
220-225	105
245-250	120
275	135
300-305	150
325-330	165
345-350	175
370-375	190
400-405	205
425-430	220
445-450	230
470-475	245
500	260

LIQUID MEASURE TO LITERS

¼	cup	=	0.06	liters
½	cup	=	0.12	liters
¾	cup	=	0.18	liters
1	cup	=	0.24	liters
1-¼	cups	=	0.3	liters
1-½	cups	=	0.36	liters
2	cups	=	0.48	liters
2-½	cups	=	0.6	liters
3	cups	=	0.72	liters
3-½	cups	=	0.84	liters
4	cups	=	0.96	liters
4-½	cups	=	1.08	liters
5	cups	=	1.2	liters
5-½	cups	=	1.32	liters

Index

Veggie-Bean Ragout, 251
Voluptuous Vegetables, 211–243

Wakame
  Cucumber-Wakame Salsa, 242–243
Walnuts
  Hearty Greens with Spiced Walnuts, 235–236
Water, 84–85
Watercress
  Crispy Tempeh with Sweet Mustard Sauce,
    265–266
  Roasted Artichoke and Turnip Salad with
    Raspberry Vinaigrette, 219–220
  Shiitake and Scallion Pâté, 227–228
  Soba with Shiitake Mushrooms and Scallions,
    207–208

Spicy Carrot Soup with Asian-Style Greens,
  175–176
Summer Hiziki Salad, 239–240
Watercress and Fried Mushroom Salad, 233–
  234
White Beans and Vegetable Soup, 180
Whites of the eyes, 43–44
Wild Rice with Hato Mugi and Vegetables, 201–
  202
Winter Squash and Carrot Puree, 222–223
Winter Squash and Millet Soup, 174–175
Wrinkles, 92–93

Ying and yang, 4–6, 19
Your Glowing Roots, 1–19
Your Glowing Skin, 79–98

From public television's award-winning
Christina Pirello,
more great ideas for living well.

Glow
A Prescription for Radiant Health and Beauty

Cook Your Way to the Life You Want

Christina Cooks
Everything You Always Wanted to Know
About Whole Foods but Were Afraid to Ask

Cooking the Whole Foods Way, Revised

This Crazy Vegan Life
A Prescription for an Endangered Species

penguin.com

T28.0208